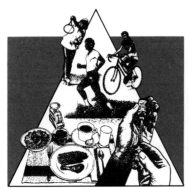

Managing Diabetes Properly

SECOND EDITION
NURSING85 BOOKS™
SPRINGHOUSE CORPORATION
SPRINGHOUSE, PENNSYLVANIA

Managing Diabetes Properly

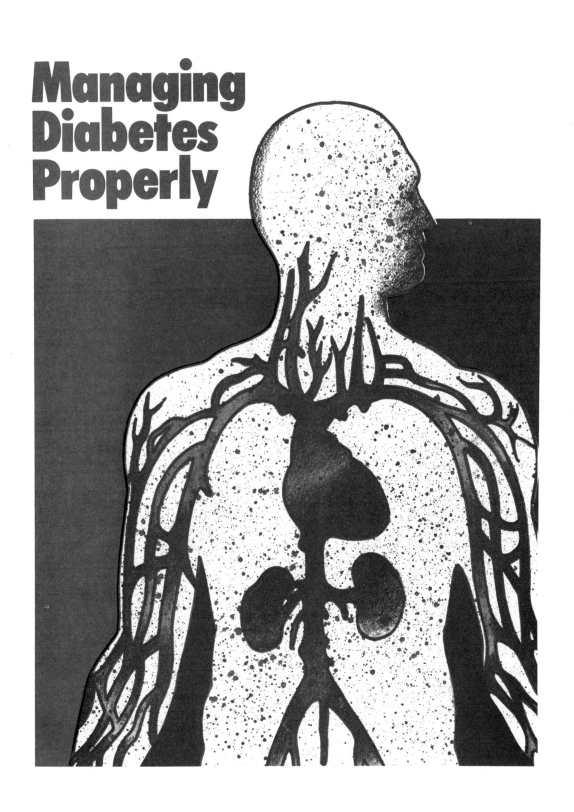

**NEW NURSING SKILLBOOK™
Series**
PROGRAM DIRECTOR
Jean Robinson

CLINICAL DIRECTOR
Barbara McVan, RN

ART DIRECTOR
John Hubbard

PROJECT MANAGER
Susan Rossi Williams

**Springhouse Corporation
Book Division**
CHAIRMAN
Eugene W. Jackson

PRESIDENT
Daniel L. Cheney

VICE-PRESIDENT AND
DIRECTOR
Timothy B. King

VICE-PRESIDENT, BOOK
OPERATIONS
Thomas A. Temple

VICE-PRESIDENT, PRODUCTION
AND PURCHASING
Bacil Guiley

Staff for this edition:
BOOK EDITOR: Patricia R. Urosevich
CLINICAL EDITOR: Barbara McVan, RN
ASSISTANT EDITOR: Jo Lennon
DESIGNER: Kathaleen Motak Singel
CONTRIBUTING DESIGNER: Lorraine Lostracco Carbo
COPY SUPERVISOR: David R. Moreau
COPY EDITORS: Traci A. Deraco, Diane M. Labus, Carolyn Mortimer, Doris
   Weinstock
EDITORIAL ASSISTANTS: Lynn C. Borders, Ellen Johnson
ILLUSTRATORS: Jack Crane, Robert Jackson
ART PRODUCTION MANAGER: Robert Perry
ARTISTS: Donald G. Knauss, Robert Miele, Sandra Sanders, Louise
   Stamper, John Walsh, Robert Wieder
TYPOGRAPHY MANAGER: David C. Kosten
TYPOGRAPHY ASSISTANTS: Ethel Halle, Diane Paluba, Nancy Wirs
SENIOR PRODUCTION MANAGER: Deborah C. Meiris
PRODUCTION MANAGER: Wilbur D. Davidson
PRODUCTION ASSISTANT: T.A. Landis
COVER ART: Brendan Riley
DIVIDER ART: John Freas

Clinical consultants for this edition:
K. Patrick Ober, MD, *Assistant Professor of Medicine, Bowman Gray School
   of Medicine, Winston-Salem, N.C.*
Diane Powers, RN, MS, *Certified Adult Nurse Practitioner, American Ge-
   riatrics and Gerontology, Inc., Albuquerque, N.M.*
Nancy S. Storz, EdD, *Nutrition Consultant, Pottstown, Pa.*

Staff for first edition:
BOOK EDITOR: Patricia S. Chaney
RESEARCHER: Avery Rome
COPY EDITOR: Patricia A. Hamilton
PRODUCTION MANAGER: Bernard Haas
PRODUCTION ASSISTANTS: David Kosten, Margie Tyson
DESIGNER: Sally Collins
ILLUSTRATORS: Jack Crane, John Freas
ART ASSISTANTS: Maggie Arnott, Owen G. Heinrich, Patricia Wertz

Library of Congress Cataloging in
Publication Data

Main entry under title:

Managing diabetes properly.
   (New Nursing Skillbook series)
   "Nursing85 books."
   Bibliography: p.
   Includes indexes.
   1. Diabetes—Nursing.
2. Diabetes in children—Nursing.
I. Series. [DNLM: 2. Diabetes Melli-
tus—nursing. WY 155 M266]
RC660.M34 1985
610.73'6   85-2701
ISBN 0-916730-69-7

Photo on page 40 courtesy of Pfizer Inc., New York.

Contents

How to help special patients

How to give in-hospital care

Contributors

Veronica F. Engle, RN, is an assistant professor in the School of Nursing, University of Wisconsin, Madison.

Leah A. Gabriel, RN, MSN, is a former clinical editor for Springhouse Corporation, Springhouse, Pa.

Catherine D. Garofano, RN, BS, works as a clinical nurse in the endocrine-metabolic unit and serves as a senior instructor in medicine at Hahnemann University Medical School and Hospital, Philadelphia.

Larry N. Gever, RPh, PharmD, is drug information manager, Springhouse Corporation, Springhouse, Pa.

Diana W. Guthrie, RN, PhD, FAAN, is a diabetes nurse specialist and associate professor at the University of Kansas School of Medicine, Wichita, and adjunct associate professor for the department of nursing, Wichita State University.

Richard A. Guthrie, MD, is professor and director of the Kansas Regional Diabetes Center of the University of Kansas School of Medicine, Wichita.

Susan Kaufmann, RN, BS, is a coordinator of teaching nurses at Joslin Diabetes Foundation in Boston.

Edwina A. McConnell, RN, MS, is an independent nurse consultant and part-time staff nurse at Madison (Wis.) General Hospital.

K. Patrick Ober, MD, is an assistant professor of medicine at Bowman Gray School of Medicine, Winston-Salem, North Carolina.

Michael L. O'Connor, MD, is associate professor of pathology and director of clinical pathology at Bowman Gray School of Medicine and North Carolina Baptist Hospital in Winston-Salem.

Judith C. Petrokas, RN, serves as a diabetes clinical nurse specializing in education at the Miami Valley Hospital in Dayton, Ohio.

Diane Powers, RN, MS, is a certified adult nurse practitioner in Albuquerque, N.M.

Joyce Schultz, RN, is a rehabilitation nurse for the Minneapolis Society for the Blind.

Delores Schumann, RN, MS, FAAN, is an assistant professor in the faculty nursing department at the University of Michigan, Flint.

Marie Williams, BA, MSW, is a supervisor of social science for the Minneapolis Society for the Blind.

Karen Witt, RN, is an assistant professor at the University of Wisconsin–Eau Claire School of Nursing.

Lawrence W. Wolfe, BSc, RPh is vice-president of Center Consultants, Inc., Blue Bell, Pa.

Advisory Board

Foreword

No matter what your nursing field, you can't overlook diabetes. Whether you work in a newborn nursery, a hospital, a nursing home, or a community agency, you'll see diabetic patients in your practice.

But your involvement with diabetes runs deeper than with most diseases. For years, nurses have used diabetes as their model when caring for someone with a chronic disease. Then, when nurses began acting as primary care givers, diabetes was one of the first chronic diseases for which they developed protocols. Today, as the emphasis of health care shifts from episodic care to prevention, nurses are becoming even more deeply involved as patient educators. In short, nurses are getting a chance to act independently in the care of diabetic patients. They're delivering primary care and teaching patients to live with and manage their disease within their own life-styles.

For all of these reasons, you may want to sharpen your skills in caring for diabetic patients, and that's why we've updated this Skillbook. Fully revised and up to the minute, it addresses itself to the basic knowledge you'll need to care for patients with diabetes, whether diabetes is their major medical problem or just an adjunct to their major medical problem. This book starts with recognition — an important first step since you are apt to be the first member of the health team to recognize the symptoms of diabetes. It thoroughly covers treatment, not only for the average diabetic but also for those who are surgical patients as well as for those who are pregnant or blind. And it covers patient education — perhaps your greatest role in caring for diabetic patients.

This New Nursing Skillbook presents the most current information on diabetes. And it builds on itself. At the end of each section, you'll find a Skillcheck that helps you synthesize all the material you've just read and apply it to your particular practice.

Diabetes doesn't have to be a problem for you; instead, it should be a nursing challenge. By developing an understanding of diabetic patients' emotional and physical needs, you can better care for them in both chronic and acute settings. It's a challenging, rewarding way to deliver nursing care.

—BARBARA CHRISTMAN ADAIR, RN, MSN
Past-President, American Association of
Diabetes Educators
Associate Professor, Medical-Surgical Nursing
Vanderbilt University, Nashville

HOW TO RECOGNIZE AND TREAT DIABETES

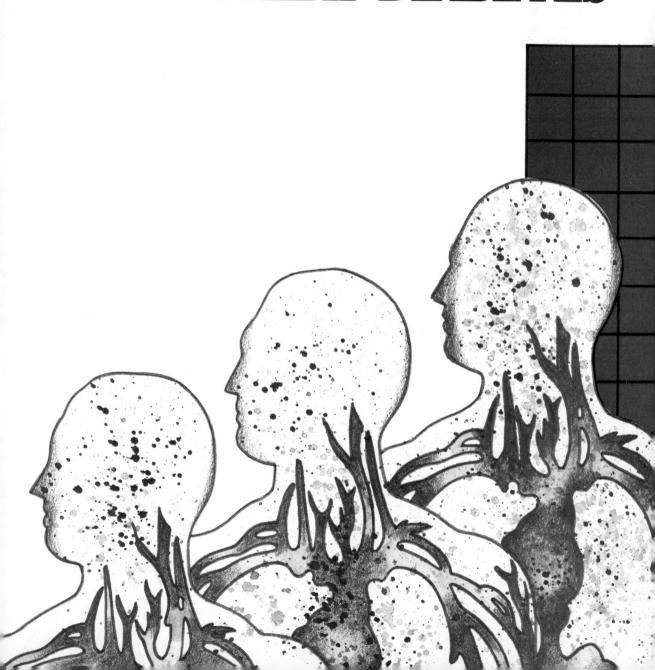

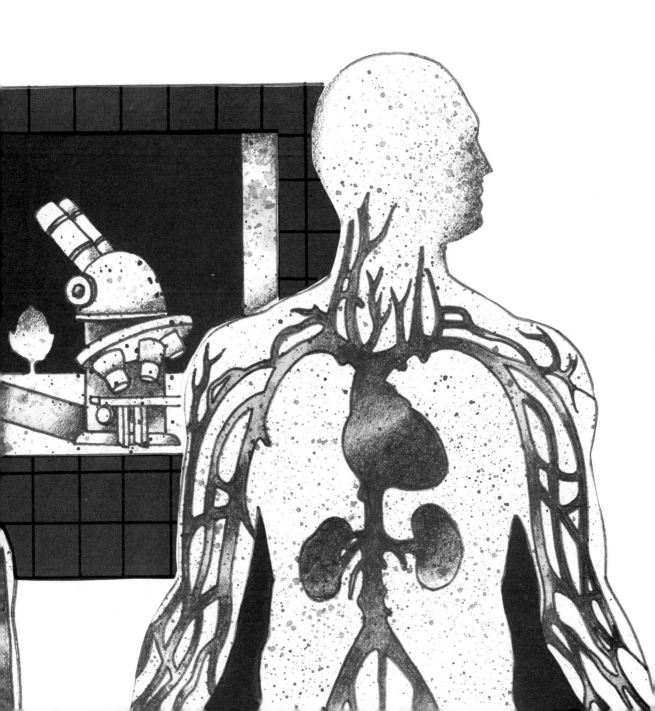

Why is the fasting blood glucose test
sometimes unreliable?

What dietary changes can you suggest to
forestall hypoglycemia?

What are the drawbacks of oral hypoglycemic
drug therapy?

What diabetic patient
would you consider a candidate for
an insulin infusion pump?

1

Diabetes:
New causes and classifications

BY LEAH A. GABRIEL, RN, MSN

JUST WHAT is diabetes? Think about it for a minute; actually take time to answer the question.

Now, examine your answer. Did you find yourself describing it in terms of metabolism? In terms of insufficient insulin and elevated blood glucose levels? If you're a typical nurse, you probably did. And technically your answer may be perfectly correct. But I wonder if it was extensive enough...if it was *practical*. Think again: Would your answer help a diabetic patient manage his disease better?

Unfortunately it's probably only a start, because nurses and most practitioners are accustomed to viewing diabetes clinically. Yet to a diabetic patient, particularly a new insulin-dependent diabetic patient, the disease is something much more fundamental — an ongoing threat to his financial status, to his life-style, and to his very life. And to give him practical help in managing his diabetes, you must approach it from *his* perspective.

That's not always easy, even if you often work with diabetic patients or are diabetic yourself. I remember one of my patients who had just learned of his diabetes and seemed very upset. Based on my experience, I immediately assumed that he was concerned about some part of his therapy. So I reviewed his diet and insulin injections over and over again.

Etiology: Who develops diabetes?

Why some people develop diabetes mellitus remains a mystery, but we do know that these factors play important roles:

• *Genetics:* While Type I diabetic patients may have a family history, they're more likely to have certain predisposing genetic patterns that help predict who will develop diabetes. Using the human leukocyte antigen (HLA) system as a genetic marker, researchers found a link between Type I diabetes and certain HLA patterns.

Although no HLA antigen pattern has been linked to Type II diabetic patients, such patients generally have a strong hereditary link.

• *Viruses:* Because viral infections may affect the pancreas of a person with a genetic predisposition to diabetes, researchers are investigating a possible link between viruses and Type I diabetes. Antibody production, which normally follows a viral infection, can attack pancreatic beta cells and lead to diabetes. One virus, Coxsackie B$_4$, is known to destroy beta cells. So far, twenty other viruses have also been linked to Type I diabetes.

• *Autoimmunity:* Because some diabetic patients develop antibodies to pancreatic islet cells, researchers believe an abnormal immune response linked to diabetes causes the body to incorrectly recognize pancreatic beta cells as foreign and destroy them. A defective HLA system can also affect the immune system and have the same destructive effect. Cyclosporine, a drug that suppresses the immune response, is being studied to determine its value in treating or reversing diabetes.

He still seemed upset. Only later did I discover why: his real concern wasn't diet and insulin therapy but rather impotence, which had been his first symptom of diabetes. Fortunately his wife finally explained his concern to me so the doctor and I could help him deal with it. If his wife hadn't intervened, though, I'm sure that man would have taken a long time to adjust to his condition — thanks to my lack of adequate information.

That story underlines what I believe is the most important precept of nursing for diabetic patients: To help a new diabetic patient cope with his diagnosis, you have to develop not only a clinical appreciation of diabetes but also a practical perspective. The balance of this book is devoted to the practical side of diabetes. When you finish reading it, you should be better able to truly help your patients manage their diabetes.

But with diabetes, as with all diseases, practice must be grounded in clinical theory. So let's get back to my original question: Just what is diabetes? To help you understand it practically, here's a brief clinical explanation.

Simply stated, diabetes is a group of disorders characterized by glucose intolerance. It's chief manifestations include alterations in the metabolism of insulin, carbohydrates, fats, and proteins and in the structure and function of blood vessels and nerves. Early signs and symptoms of the disease stem from metabolic disorders; later complications stem from vascular and nervous system disorders.

Blood glucose control

You probably know that glucose (a carbohydrate) is an efficient, readily available energy source. (How many times have you eaten a candy bar for a quick pick-me-up?) But did you know that the body relies on glucose as its *chief* fuel? That's right: Even though fat and protein also provide energy, glucose is the fuel that your body needs most. In particular, it's the only energy source that yields enough energy to maintain function of the brain — which can't function without it.

But the beneficial effects of glucose occur only when the body's glucose levels stay within a fairly narrow range. To achieve this, several hormones — primarily insulin and glucagon — regulate glucose levels in blood and tissues. Insulin and glucagon work together, via feedback mechanisms, to maintain blood glucose levels within a normal range so that

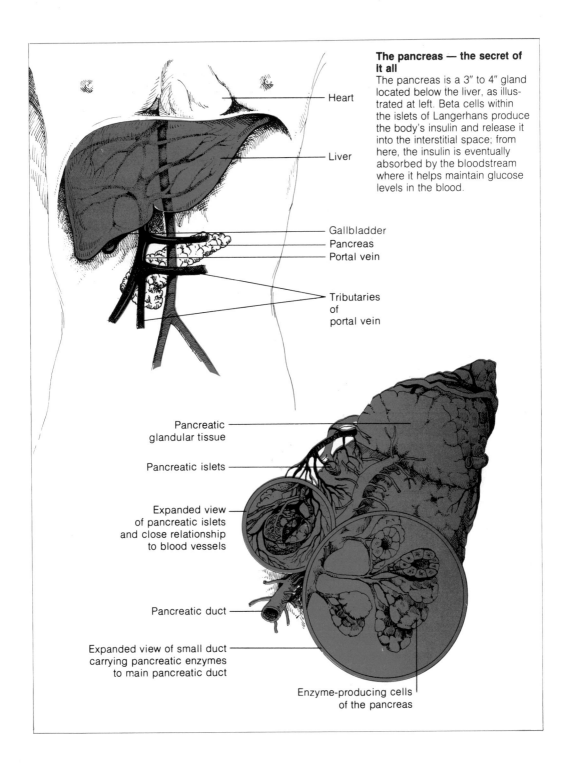

Heart

Liver

The pancreas — the secret of it all
The pancreas is a 3″ to 4″ gland located below the liver, as illustrated at left. Beta cells within the islets of Langerhans produce the body's insulin and release it into the interstitial space; from here, the insulin is eventually absorbed by the bloodstream where it helps maintain glucose levels in the blood.

Gallbladder
Pancreas
Portal vein

Tributaries
of
portal vein

Pancreatic
glandular tissue

Pancreatic islets

Expanded view
of pancreatic islets
and close relationship
to blood vessels

Pancreatic duct

Expanded view of small duct
carrying pancreatic enzymes
to main pancreatic duct

Enzyme-producing cells
of the pancreas

Classifying diabetes

Because diabetes mellitus is now believed to be a cluster of disorders, the National Institutes of Health, National Diabetes Data Group has reclassified diabetes as follows:

DIABETES MELLITUS
• Type I, insulin-dependent diabetes mellitus (IDDM), was formerly known as "juvenile-onset" or "brittle" diabetes. Type I can strike at any age, although most patients are young. All Type I diabetic patients require insulin replacement for life.
• Type II, non-insulin-dependent diabetes mellitus (NIDDM), formerly known as "adult-onset" or "stable" diabetes, accounts for about 90% of all diabetic patients. Most Type II diabetic patients are over age 40 and obese.
• Other types, formerly known as "secondary diabetes," include several subcategories of conditions known or suspected to cause diabetes. These include pancreatic, hormonal, and drug-induced causes, abnormalities of cellular receptor sites, and certain genetic syndromes.

GESTATIONAL DIABETES
Gestational diabetes develops during pregnancy and increases the risk of perinatal complications. Many of these patients will later develop another form of diabetes. If their blood glucose levels remain elevated following pregnancy, they are then reclassified into another diabetes category.

IMPAIRED GLUCOSE TOLERANCE (IGT)
IGT occurs in patients who have normal or slightly elevated fasting blood glucose levels but have abnormal glucose tolerance tests. Most of these patients are asymptomatic, and many do not develop diabetes.

cells' metabolic needs are met. In effect, secretion of one stimulates secretion of the other as the blood glucose level is correspondingly raised or lowered.

Insulin. Following ingestion of a carbohydrate, glucose is absorbed into the bloodstream, elevating the blood glucose level. In response, the pancreatic beta cells (in the islets of Langerhans) secrete insulin, which binds to the receptors on insulin-dependent cells (which make up most of the body) and allows them to absorb the extra glucose. If this initial response reduces the blood glucose level to normal, no more insulin is secreted. But if the blood glucose level remains elevated after the initial response, the beta cells make and release more insulin. Either way, the body's glucose levels usually return to a normal range within 2 hours after ingestion of a high-carbohydrate meal.

Besides allowing cells to absorb excess glucose from the bloodstream, insulin acts in other ways to lower blood glucose levels and to facilitate anabolism. Here are some of the most important ways insulin benefits a Type I diabetic patient:
• It aids in the storage of glucose as glycogen — a process called glycogenesis — and so inhibits breakdown of glycogen to glucose (glycogenolysis).
• It prevents breakdown of amino acids to glucose (gluconeogenesis) in the liver by suppressing the deamidization of the amino acid, alanine.
• It helps prevent fat cell storage (fat cells store glucose).

Glucagon. To prevent blood glucose levels from dropping too low and to provide glucose during times of exercise and fasting (between meals), the alpha cells of the pancreas secrete the hormone glucagon, which — in contrast to insulin — *raises* blood glucose levels. Glucagon works by signaling the liver to convert glycogen to glucose and to convert proteins to amino acids — which are further broken down into glucose. This process also promotes the breakdown of fats to fatty acids and glycerol (which contributes to the total amount of available glucose).

Other hormones. Besides insulin and glucagon, hormones that influence blood glucose levels include:
• catecholamines (epinephrine and norepinephrine), which are secreted by the adrenal medulla and the sympathetic nervous system. These hormones *raise* blood glucose levels by stimulating glycogenolysis, by inhibiting insulin release, and

by facilitating breakdown of free fatty acids.

• glucocorticoids, secreted from the adrenal cortex. These hormones enhance gluconeogenesis.

• growth hormone (somatotropin), secreted from the anterior pituitary gland. In response to stress, periods of growth, or prolonged hypoglycemia, increased secretion of growth hormone slows the cells' use of glucose and increases the mobilization of fats for energy.

• somatostatin, secreted by the pancreas, and gastrin, secreted by the GI tract. Somatostatin *inhibits* either insulin or glucagon secretion, according to blood glucose levels, whereas gastrin, *stimulates* either process.

• several intestinal hormones, secreted during digestion. These indirectly influence blood glucose levels—for example, gastric inhibitory peptide stimulates insulin secretion.

Altered metabolism in diabetes
In a patient with diabetes, hormonal regulation of blood glucose levels goes awry, altering carbohydrate, protein, and fat metabolism. How much these processes are altered depends on the patient's degree of insulin deficiency or insulin resistance (inability to use the insulin he has — for example, if his cells lack adequate numbers of insulin receptors). Let's look at the metabolic changes that occur in both Type I and Type II diabetic patients. (See the marginalia opposite, the chart on page 19, and the information on page 20.)

Carbohydrates. Without insulin, or if insulin is present but can't be used (insulin resistance), cells can't store glucose or use it as fuel for energy. The result? Hyperglycemia. Here's what happens:

When *insufficient* insulin is present to inhibit glycogenolysis, the liver produces glucose from glycogen. Certain hormones, such as gastrin, also increase blood glucose levels, stimulating alpha cells to secrete glucagon. If these two processes balance out, the body may not make extra glucose because some cellular needs are being met. But if no insulin is present, or if insulin is deficient, the body overproduces glucose, leading to hyperglycemia.

Fats. Without insulin, fats are converted to free fatty acids and so they float freely in the bloodstream. On reaching the liver, they're metabolized. This leads to the production of ketone bodies, which accumulate (when compensatory mechanisms

Statistical risk
Patients with a previous abnormality of glucose tolerance (sometimes called PreVAGT) have had abnormal glucose tolerance tests or have had hyperglycemia in the past but have reverted to normal. This condition is often associated with stress, such as from an infection.

Patients with a potential for abnormal glucose tolerance (sometimes called PotAGT) have normal glucose test results but later develop diabetes. Patients in this category who are most likely to develop diabetes have two parents or an identical twin with diabetes.

Other patients at risk include those who are obese and women who deliver babies weighing over 9 lb. Unfortunately, because no screening test for diabetes is now available that can diagnose the disease before onset of hyperglycemia or finding of an abnormal glucose tolerance test, these patients can't be identified. However, with recent breakthroughs in genetics, some expensive new tests are available that will improve the chances of early diagnosis.

fail) and lead to ketoacidosis.

Protein. Without protein, cell growth and cell repair don't take place: protein wasting accompanies severe insulin deficiency and causes accumulation of amino acids in the bloodstream. Gluconeogenesis also occurs because of the lack of insulin's inhibitory effect.

Clinical effects

In a diabetic patient, the metabolic alterations described above cause depletion of cells' energy stores and subsequent cell starvation. Depletion of protein and fat stimulates the patient's appetite (polyphagia) as his body tries to take in the nutrients necessary to reverse the catabolic state.

As his blood glucose level rises, it increases plasma osmotic pressure, drawing water out of cells. When the renal threshold for glucose is exceeded, glycosuria results, then polyuria as glucose pulls water with it. His thirst increases, too (polydipsia) — a compensatory mechanism for restoring fluid lost through the kidneys and cells. He may require fluid replacement to prevent dehydration.

Of course, hyperglycemia is the clinical hallmark of diabetes. But, long before such conclusive signs of diabetes appear, other warning signs may arise.

Common early warning signals involve the skin, in the form of shin spots, recurrent infections, or recalcitrant fungal infections.

• Shin spots, which occur more often in men than in women, may develop from a blow on the shin. A distinct brown spot about the size of a penny appears on the front of the shin.

• Recurrent infections include boils, carbuncles, and furuncles. Although these appear most often on the posterior neck, they can develop anywhere on the body.

• Recalcitrant fungal infections develop between toes or in nail beds. True, nondiabetic patients may develop the same infections. But people prone to diabetes seem particularly susceptible to them.

Strangely enough, hypoglycemia, which is the direct opposite of diabetes, also can be a sign of impending hyperglycemia or early diabetes in an adult. Usually the symptoms of hypoglycemia (tremors, sweating, headache, fatigue, and faintness) appear 3 to 5 hours after the person has eaten. What happens is this: After eating a glucose load, the patient has a sluggish insulin response. So, for the first couple of hours after eating, his blood glucose level is quite high. In response to the excessive glucose, his pancreas finally sends forth an excessive dose of insulin, which eventually lowers the glucose level well below normal.

Finally, many of the complications of diabetes (see Chapter 10) may develop before the diabetes itself is apparent. These early warnings include eye changes, kidney dysfunction, numbness and tingling in the feet or legs, vascular disease, and hardening of the arteries.

If any of these early warning signs appears, particularly any combination of them, you should advise a patient to have his blood glucose levels checked.

Type I differences

Although it can occur at any age, Type I diabetes usually

Characteristics of Type I and Type II Diabetes		
CHARACTERISTIC	TYPE I	TYPE II
Former name	• Juvenile-onset diabetes • Brittle diabetes	• Adult-onset diabetes • Stable diabetes
Age at onset	• Usually under age 40	• Usually over age 40
Type of onset	• Abrupt	• Gradual
Percentage of diabetic patients in category	• 10%	• 90%
Obesity incidence	• Usually absent	• Present in 80% of patients
Physiologic changes	• Beta cell destruction • Inadequate insulin secretion • Inability of beta cell to secrete or release insulin • Abnormal insulin molecule • Destruction of insulin before it reaches target cell • Insulin binding in serum	• Deficiency of insulin receptors • Abnormal receptor • Antibodies to receptor • Cell membrane defects • Intracellular defects that prohibit cell from using glucose • Impaired release of insulin
Ketoacidosis incidence	• More likely to develop	• Less likely to develop if ketosis occurs; usually related to stress, such as from rapid weight loss
Endogenous insulin production	• Absent	• Present

Be optimistic!
Perhaps what the diabetic patient needs most is your encouragement and optimism. Throughout your teaching, emphasize that, with judicious self-care, he can live a nearly normal life. That bit of optimism, combined with your realistic instructions, will help him learn to handle his condition with practicality and wisdom.

develops during childhood or puberty. Because its hallmark is a total lack of insulin, it comes with stunning swiftness. Without any insulin, the child may go into diabetic ketoacidosis (DKA) — sometimes the first clue to the child's disease. Because Type I diabetic patients must rely totally on exogenous insulin, they must get prompt treatment to control their condition. And because their condition is more serious and erratic than a Type II diabetic patient's, they're more prone to ketoacidosis, hypoglycemia, and hyperglycemic hyperosmolar nonketotic coma (HHNC).

Type II differences

You may recall that Type II diabetic patients do produce some insulin; the problem is either insufficient quantities of it or resistance to it. Type II diabetic patients generally *don't* develop ketoacidosis, because they're able to use some glucose (but not all of it) and so prevent fat breakdown. However, because they don't have enough insulin to handle all the glucose, hyperglycemia results. Some Type II diabetic patients, however, may be asymptomatic even with severely elevated blood glucose levels.

Obese patients with insulin resistance (the majority of diabetic patients) appear to have a deficiency of cellular insulin receptors. Usually weight reduction reverses this deficiency and normalizes the patient's blood glucose level.

In some Type II diabetic patients, the pancreas produces excess insulin to lower blood glucose levels. But because these patients have fewer cellular receptor sites (the more insulin released, the fewer receptor sites available) to bind insulin, they can't use this excess insulin and it has no effect. So they remain hyperglycemic.

Remember these important points when teaching your patient about the causes of diabetes:
1. Diabetes is a group of disorders characterized by glucose intolerance.
2. Insulin and glucagon work together to maintain normal blood glucose levels.
3. Genetics, viral infections, and autoimmunity may play a role in the etiology of diabetes.

2

Confirming suspicions with laboratory tests

BY MICHAEL L. O'CONNOR, MD

ALTHOUGH DIABETES SCREENING and diagnostic tests are simple procedures that give accurate results when done correctly, they can be misleading if the patient isn't properly prepared. That's where you come in. Since you're in the best position to monitor the patient's preparation, you can play an important role in determining the tests' reliability.

Screening tests for diabetes measure glucose in either urine or blood. Of these, the urine glucose measurement is simpler, requiring no advance preparation. A reagent strip is dipped into the urine specimen (or a Clinitest tablet is mixed with urine in a test tube). The resulting color indicates the glucose concentration. But this test can diagnose only Type I, or insulin-dependent, diabetes. This is because the blood glucose concentration must exceed 140 mg/dl — well above the normal levels and the levels associated with other types of diabetes — before glucose will spill over into urine.

The fasting blood glucose test, which should be done between 7 a.m. and 12 noon, is the screening tool of choice. Be sure to advise a patient scheduled for this test not to eat or take any medications (except with the doctor's permission) for 10 hours before the test.

Some doctors prefer a 1- or 2-hour postprandial glucose test to diagnose patients with diabetes. For this test, the patient

Diseases that affect glucose tolerance

Patients recovering from severe illnesses or surgery should have glucose tolerance tests postponed. Here are some of the effects of some diseases:

- *Peripheral resistance to insulin* caused by diseases requiring prolonged bed rest, such as chronic neuromuscular disorders and hip fractures
- *Sluggish insulin response* caused by acute starvation states or malnutrition
- *Glucose intolerance* caused by acromegaly, Cushing's syndrome, or potassium loss
- *Carbohydrate intolerance* caused by pheochromocytoma or hyperthyroidism

eats a meal of about 100 g of carbohydrates (the glucose load) after an overnight fast. Then, 1 or 2 hours later, the blood sample is drawn.

In some hospitals, nurses draw the samples and send them to the laboratory for analysis, while in others the patient is sent to the laboratory for the procedure. Whichever is the policy in your hospital, you are responsible for seeing that the patient fasts and eats adequately at the appropriate times.

If the fasting blood glucose test reveals a glucose level of 140 mg/dl or above, or if a 1- or 2-hour postprandial glucose test yields glucose levels above 200 mg/dl or above 160 mg/dl, respectively, the patient probably has diabetes; an oral glucose tolerance test (OGTT) wouldn't tell you much more. But if the results of the screening test are ambiguous or indicate probable diabetes (see chart on opposite page), the patient should have an OGTT to confirm the diagnosis.

Patients at higher risk for diabetes than the general population are commonly given the OGTT instead of a screening test. These patients include:

- those with a family history of diabetes
- obese patients
- those with transitory glycosuria or nondiagnostic hyperglycemia, especially during the course of pregnancy, surgical procedures, trauma, emotional stress, myocardial infarction, cerebrovascular accident, or administration of adrenal steroids
- those with unexplained episodes of hypoglycemia
- women who have delivered large babies or have had pregnancies resulting in abortions, premature labor, stillbirths, or neonatal deaths
- those with unexplained neuropathy, retinopathy, nephropathy, or peripheral vascular disease.

Generally, the diagnostic OGTT should be performed only on ambulatory patients who are not acutely ill or recovering from major surgery or acute illness. If an ill person is overtly diabetic, the 2-hour postprandial screening test will detect the diabetes. If it doesn't, the diagnostic test should be delayed until his metabolism has returned to normal — usually when he is ambulatory.

Preparing your patient

Patient preparation for the OGTT is most important. Improper

Serum Glucose		
1-HOUR POSTPRANDIAL	2-HOUR POSTPRANDIAL	DIAGNOSIS
Below 150 mg/dl	Below 120 mg/dl	Normal
150 to 185 mg/dl	120 to 140 mg/dl	Ambiguous
186 to 200 mg/dl	141 to 160 mg/dl	Probable diabetes
Over 200 mg/dl	Over 160 mg/dl	Diabetes

preparation is probably the greatest source of error in diabetes testing.

Diet. Be sure the patient is on a normal diet with an intake of at least 300 g of carbohydrates per day for 3 days preceding the test. When you describe the test procedure to the patient, stress the importance of his eating the loading diet. You can suggest that the patient eat his normal diet *plus* high-carbohydrate snacks at midmorning, midafternoon, and bedtime. Make the following exceptions, though: If the patient is grossly overweight and following a 300-g/day carbohydrate reducing diet, don't put him on the 3-day preparatory diet. If the patient has been anorexic or eating poorly, put him on a preparatory diet for 7 days.

Medication. See that all drugs are discontinued for at least 3 days before the test. (But be sure to check with the patient's doctor before doing so.) If a patient is on oral contraceptives, have her omit them for one cycle, if possible.

Fasting period. See that the patient has no food for at least 10 but not more than 16 hours preceding the test. He may have water, however.

Miscellaneous restrictions. Be sure that the patient avoids drinking coffee, smoking, and doing any unusual physical exercise for at least 8 hours before and during the test.

Again, depending on your hospital's policy, you may collect the specimens yourself or send the patient to the laboratory for the test. If the patient is to have the test done in the laboratory, you should see that he is dressed warmly and that he has something to occupy his time during the test (for example, reading material, puzzles or games, or handiwork).

The test should be conducted between 7 a.m. and 12 noon, with the fasting specimens (blood and urine) taken between 7 a.m. and 9 a.m. If it's necessary that the patient be weighed before the test, be sure you actually weigh him — don't just ask him his weight.

Drugs that affect glucose tolerance
Some medications elevate blood glucose levels; others depress it. Here are some effects to keep in mind when you're assessing a patient's test results.
Elevate glucose levels: diazoxide (Hyperstat), nicotinic acid (niacin), oral contraceptives containing mestranol (Enovid, Norinyl, Ortho-Novum, Ovulen), phenytoin (Dilantin), systemic glucocorticoids, and thiazides and other potassium-depleting diuretics
Depress glucose levels: alcohol, salicylates (chronic high dosage)

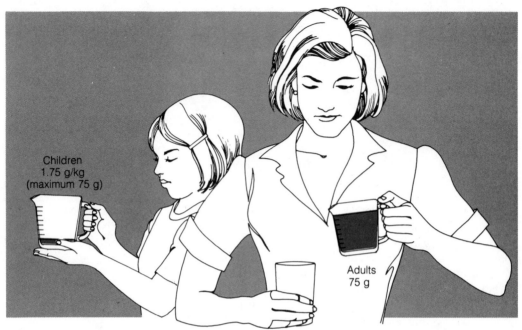

Children
1.75 g/kg
(maximum 75 g)

Adults
75 g

How much glucose should you give?

The loading dose of oral glucose, usually a 25% solution, must be administered over several minutes in a dosage appropriate to the patient's age and, for some patients, body size.

If you're doing the test yourself, administer the oral glucose (loading dose) over several minutes. Usually, a 25% glucose solution flavored with noncaloric cola, orange, or lemon is given in the quantities shown in the above illustration.

After the patient's fast, draw an antecubital venous blood specimen. If your patient's a child, perform a fingerstick to obtain capillary blood. Note "time zero" (when the patient starts drinking the glucose). Draw additional blood specimens exactly 60, 90, 120, and 180 minutes after time zero (and at 240 and 300 minutes after for a 5-hour test). A urine specimen may also be requested.

You may also be asked to collect simultaneous urine specimens. Although not required for the interpretation of the test, they give information about the patient's renal glucose threshold, which is potentially useful in adjusting insulin dosage if such therapy is required.

If whole blood, without preservatives, is obtained, the specimens must be analyzed within ½ hour after collection. So, you must deliver the specimens, properly labeled, promptly to the laboratory. (If this is impossible, separate the serum as soon as the blood is clotted.) Your laboratory may suggest that you collect the specimens in fluoride tubes, which make glucose assays valid for up to 48 hours.

If the patient vomits the ingested glucose during the first

hour, the results will be invalidated, so you should cancel the test at once and reschedule it for another day.

Other diagnostic tests

To confirm a diagnosis of probable diabetes, the doctor may order the plasma insulin or glycosylated hemoglobin test.

Plasma insulin test: This test is used to determine if the patient has insulin deficiency or is insulin-resistant. It may also be done to help determine the cause of hypoglycemia.

Because an increase in plasma glucose increases insulin secretion, two blood specimens — one for plasma insulin and one for blood glucose—must be drawn, and the results must be compared.

Serum insulin levels must be interpreted in relation to the simultaneous serum glucose concentration. While most diabetic patients will have low insulin levels, even in the presence of high glucose, some obese insulin-resistant diabetic patients will have normal levels. Make sure the patient is relaxed before drawing the blood sample, because anxiety or stress may affect his insulin level.

Glycosylated hemoglobin test: Unlike the serum glucose test that reflects glucose regulation at only one moment in time, the fraction of hemoglobin that has become glycosylated (irreversibly chemically bonded with glucose molecules) reflects the average plasma glucose concentration over the life span (120 days) of the erythrocytes. Thus the glycosylated hemoglobin test is a valuable aid in monitoring the long-term adequacy of glucose regulation of diabetic patients. The test is typically ordered about every 6 to 8 weeks to monitor severely diabetic patients. Depending on the laboratory's test method, a glycosylated hemoglobin fraction of 8% or less is normal; diabetic patients average about 12%, with those in good control approaching the normal range and those in poor control being above 12%. The test is done on a standard venipuncture blood specimen collected in a 5-ml lavender-top tube (same tube as used for the CBC in hematology). No special handling is required.

When the test is completed, see that the patient gets something to eat.

A variety of criteria for interpreting the test data are in use, and most results will fall in the clearly normal or clearly diabetic range. These criteria were established by various in-

Glucose tolerance test curves
This chart illustrates glucose tolerance test curves for diabetic, impaired glucose tolerance, and normal adult patients.

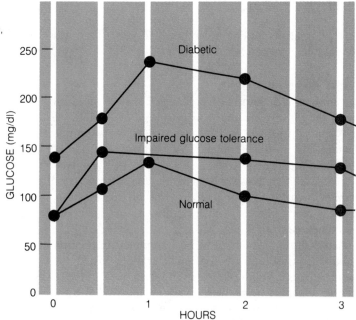

vestigators so that patients could be classified as either diabetic or nondiabetic in various research protocols. But for the individual patient, such sharp classification is somewhat artificial, so the doctor must judge his overall clinical condition to determine what follow-up or diagnosis is appropriate.

To interpret a patient's test results you should know your hospital's normal values for the OGTT and whether the test was carried out and completed as planned. The above graph will help you to make a general interpretation of the test results.

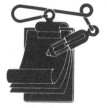

Remember these important points about laboratory tests:
1. Conduct diagnostic blood glucose tests between 7 a.m. and 12 noon.
2. Advise a patient scheduled for a fasting blood glucose test not to eat or take medication for 10 hours (an overnight fast) before testing.
3. Suspect diabetes when a decrease in the plasma insulin level corresponds to an increase in the plasma glucose level.
4. Consider two fasting blood glucose levels of 140 mg/dl or above a positive indication of diabetes.
5. Expect results of the glycosylated hemoglobin test to indicate the patient's approximate daily glucose level.

3

Diet:
Enforcing the sine qua non

BY SUSAN KAUFMANN, RN, BS

WHETHER A DIABETIC patient is Type I (insulin-dependent) or Type II (non-insulin-dependent), severely diabetic or moderately diabetic...he's sure to need one type of therapy — diet. Because diet is the sine qua non of diabetic therapy. Controlled intake of carbohydrates, fat, and protein — weighed against medications and exercise — keeps a patient balanced on that tightrope between hyperglycemia and hypoglycemia, diabetic coma and insulin shock. And recent research indicates that patients with good control of their diabetes have fewer complications.

Unfortunately, though, getting a diabetic patient to stick to a diet isn't simple. The usual litany of negatives that we give diabetic patients as a diet plan — "No desserts, no sugar in your coffee, no sporadic snacks" — hardly encourages cooperation. To encourage cooperation, you have to make the diet plan realistic for each patient's life-style. We've tried the realistic approach at the Joslin Clinic and have found it often improves initial compliance. Of course, to guarantee continued compliance, you've got to continue seeing each patient regularly and frequently. But a realistic diet-setting technique can help you handle the frustrations of initial diet instructions. The technique described in this chapter is based on our program, which applies primarily to adults. Chapter 14 suggests a few dietary modifications for diabetic children.

The problem of fat
Being overweight jeopardizes
the life of a diabetic patient. If he
is 5% to 14% overweight, he
runs twice the risk of death of a
diabetic patient at ideal weight;
15% to 24% overweight, four
times the risk; and 25% or more
overweight, ten times the risk.

Tailoring objectives

Your therapeutic goals should be no different from those recommended by most textbooks. You should plan programs to
help patients:
- reach and maintain ideal weight
- maintain proper nutrition
- assist in controlling their diabetes
- assist in preventing and controlling short-term and long-
term complications.

The diet, though, should be tailored to the patient's specific
life-style.

To really get to know each new patient and his life-style, we
invite him for a week-long course at our diabetic treatment
unit. Throughout the week, the unit's doctors give classes
in the morning, and we teaching nurses give classes in the
afternoon. We encourage the patient to attend both sessions
and to come to us for private instruction to supplement or
clarify classroom material. We also provide diet instruction
both in class and individually. But the unit's dietitian
further explains our instructions and consults patients with complicated dietary restrictions, such as gluten-free or lactose-free
diets.

Throughout the week, we also ask the patient to critique his
diet over and over, so we can modify it to make it realistic. In
this way, he has some say in setting his dietary goals and maintaining his diabetic control. And by the end of the week, we're
able to discharge him with a diet that he understands and that is
tailored to his needs.

Begin where the patient is

To establish a dietary starting point during any instruction course,
you should open by asking simple questions: "Why are you
here? What would you like to know?"

If the patient says he's having difficulty with hypoglycemic
episodes, begin there. Once you work out a dietary solution to
that problem, you may go into gourmet meal planning — if
that's what he wants. Your point, always, is to stress the
patient's objectives, to gear your instruction to what *he* wants to
know.

Early during your conversation, also determine the patient's life-style — the kind, amount, and usual times of his

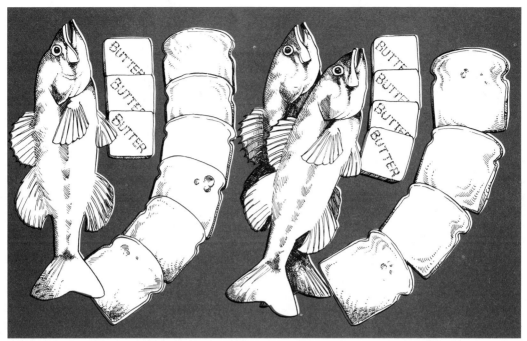

activity; his illnesses or other stresses; the type of insulin he takes and his body's response to it.

Then give him a "test" diet as a starting point.

You may follow the American Diabetes Association's diet (see pages 210 to 213). But you may make some modifications. We base the actual number of calories that a diabetic patient requires on his ideal body weight and on his level of activity:

20 calories/kg ideal weight = caloric intake for weight loss
30 calories/kg ideal weight = caloric intake for maintenance
40 calories/kg ideal weight = caloric intake for increased activity or weight gain.

The ADA suggests that 50% to 60% of these calories be consumed as carbohydrates, 10% to 15% as protein, and 30% to 35% as fat. But we generally stick to a 40-20-40 formula unless the patient has renal failure, elevated lipid levels, or other medical problems. We feel that diabetic patients don't tolerate the higher level of carbohydrates as well as they do the lower level.

Our substitution list also resembles the ADA's exchange list, with four exceptions.

First, instead of one fruit list, we provide two — small

What's for dinner?
The diet of the American Diabetes Association recommends that 60% of all calories consumed be carbohydrates, 10% be protein, and 30% be fat. The Joslin Clinic diet observes the same categories in different quantities: 40-20-40. Check with the doctor to see which diet is best for your patient.

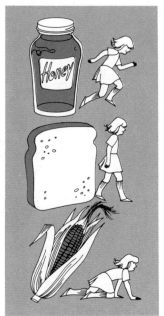

Understand carbohydrates before giving them

In giving carbohydrates to prevent hypoglycemia or to treat insulin shock, remember the following analogies:

- Sugar enters the blood as fast as a child runs.
- Starch enters the blood as fast as a child walks.
- Starch in vegetables enters the blood as fast as a child crawls.

To forestall hypoglycemia, you should suggest slower-acting starches for afternoon or evening snacks. To treat insulin shock, you should administer fast-acting sugars.

fruits and medium fruits. Small fruits can be interchanged with cookies, pretzels, and crackers; medium fruits can be interchanged with anything on the bread list.

Second, like the ADA we forbid concentrated sweets. But unlike the ADA we allow ice cream occasionally — at most once a week, unless there is some overriding reason for more, such as excessive exercise.

Third, we break down our vegetable list into 3% and 6% categories instead of using the vegetable categories designated by the ADA. We think this terminology helps the patient remember the carbohydrate content of the vegetables and reemphasizes the need to monitor intake of carbohydrates, protein, and fats.

Fourth, unless a patient is unusually inactive or the time between meals is unusually short, we generally don't recommend fruits for between-meal snacks. The reason is that we've found some fruits metabolize quickly and don't always prevent hypoglycemia. Usually we suggest slowly metabolized carbohydrates, such as bread or crackers, followed by a protein, such as a slice of cheese or peanut butter, for more "staying power." Most patients on a single dose of intermediate insulin (NPH) need only a midafternoon and evening snack, unless the time between breakfast and lunch is unusually long. More active patients generally need a midmorning snack, too.

If we're working with a patient who frequents fast-food restaurants and snacks on junk food, we give him a breakdown of the carbohydrate, protein, and fat content in these foods. (See chart on opposite page.)

Compromising for consistency

Does all this mean that, when a patient leaves your diet instruction course, he should leave with a rigid written diet of basics and substitutions — and with the admonition to "stick to it"? No. You should give written instructions — tailored, of course, to the patient's individual needs (don't use preprinted form diets). But don't insist that he stick to it "or else."

Even though we devise a realistic diet plan for each patient, we realize that he may deviate from it. Some patients just can't break lifelong habits, even though they understand why they should; others find they can't restructure their daily lives to

Nutrient composition of General Mills snacks										
	BOWS		BUGLES		BUTTONS		DAISYS		WHISTLES	
	100 g	½ oz	100 g	½ oz	100 g	½ oz	100 g	½ oz	100 g	½ oz
No. of pieces	152	22	104	15	339	48	198	28	120	17
Protein (g)	5.51	0.8	5.63	0.8	10.3	1.4	6.53	0.9	9.28	1.3
Fat (g)	37.5	5.3	37.4	5.3	28.1	4	23.5	3.3	26.5	3.8
Carbohydrate (g)	52.5	7.5	52.5	7.5	54.7	7.8	61.8	8.8	56.1	8

Nutrient composition of McDonald's foods						
	EGG McMUFFIN 126.7 g	HAM-BURGER 96.8 g	CHEESE-BURGER 110.9 g	¼-lb HAM-BURGER 156.8 g	¼-lb CHEESE-BURGER 186.2 g	BIG MAC 183.4 g
Protein (g)	17.6	13.0	16.1	26.5	31.4	26.2
Fat (g)	11.3	9.6	13.9	19.3	27.7	31.9
Carbohydrate (g)	35.2	27.8	30.0	33.4	36.3	41.2
Exchanges	2½ bread 1½ meat 1 fat	2 bread 1 meat 1 fat	2 bread 2 meat 1 fat	2 bread 3 meat 1 fat	2 bread 4 meat 2 fat	3 bread 3 meat 4 fat

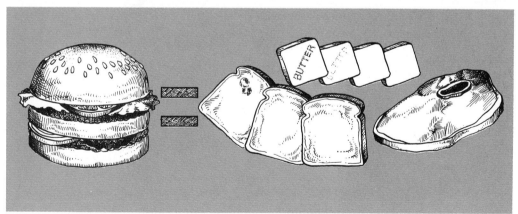

accommodate their discharge diet. So, we encourage each patient to keep in touch and to let us know if he encounters any problems with his diet. Our objective, we assure patients, is to devise a diet they can live with.

Recently, for instance, Jan, a 19-year-old college student, came to the clinic for help with midafternoon insulin reactions.

Choosing carbohydrates carefully

To improve the diabetic diet, several diabetes associations are recommending that patients reduce fat in their diets and substitute more foods from the carbohydrate group to make up the difference in calories. (Most dietitians recommend carbohydrates make up 50% of total calories consumed.) However, this requirement may pose a problem to the diabetic patient who needs to choose carbohydrates that will not cause rapid fluctuations in postprandial blood glucose levels.

Consequently, investigators are trying to categorize carbohydrates according to the serum glucose level each produces after ingestion. A rating, called the glycemic index, is assigned to each food. Foods with a low index don't cause rapid increases in serum glucose levels, while those with higher glycemic indexes do.

Although still experimental, the index could help patients select the proper carbohydrates that may minimize increases in blood glucose levels and also adapt their diets to any ethnic or personal food preferences. Most studies tested 50 g of each carbohydrate, comparing its effect with the same quantity of white bread. (White bread was used as a standard and given a rating of 100.)

Although more testing is needed, early tests have yielded surprising results. For example, researchers found that grinding rice enhanced it's glycemic effect. Pasta caused a smaller rise in postprandial blood glucose levels than bread, although both foods have a similar nutrient composition. Legumes have also produced a decreased fluctuation.

Using the Glycemic Index to Categorize Foods

FOOD	INDEX	FOOD	INDEX
Bread:		**Dried legumes:**	
Rye crisp	95	Baked beans	60
White bread	100	(canned)	
Wholegrain rye	58	Butter beans	52
Wholemeal (wheat)	99	Chick peas	49
		Dried green peas	56
Biscuits:		Haricot beans	45
Oatmeal	78	Kidney beans	54
Rich tea	80	Red lentils	43
Water	91	Soya beans	20
		(canned)	
Breakfast cereals:		Soya beans (dried)	22
All-Bran	73		
Cornflakes	119	**Fruit:**	
Muesli	96	Apple	53
Porridge oats (oat-	85	Banana	79
meal)		Cherries	32
Shredded wheat	97	Grapefruit	36
		Grapes	62
Cereal products:		Orange	66
Buckwheat	74	Orange juice	67
Millet	103	Peach	40
Rice (brown)	96	Pear	47
Rice (white)	83	Plum	34
Spaghetti (white)	66	Raisins	93
Spaghetti (whole-	61		
wheat)		**Root vegetables:**	
Sweetcorn (corn-	87	Potato (instant)	116
meal)		Potato (new,	81
		boiled)	
Dairy products:		Potato (Russet,	135
Ice cream	52	baked)	
Skim milk	46	Potato (sweet)	70
Whole milk	49	Yam	74
Yogurt	52		
		Sugars:	
		Fructose	30
		Glucose	138
		Honey	126
		Maltose	152
		Sucrose	86
		Vegetables:	
		Peas (frozen)	74

Adapted from Jenkins, D.J.A., et al., "The Glycaemic Response to Carbohydrate Foods," *Lancet* 2(8399):389, 1984, with permission of the publisher.

She was taking 50 units of NPH insulin and had a fasting blood glucose level of 65 (normal nondiabetic range 60 to 100). Lowering her insulin to 40 units partially solved the problem, but when we took her diet history, we uncovered another problem. She never ate between meals. Her reason: "I don't want to gain weight."

Since Jan was very slender — in fact, underweight — we suggested that she eat a package of peanut butter Nabs in the afternoon. She firmly refused, saying she didn't want to add any calories to her diet. Rather than insisting she do it our way — and probably not having her cooperate — we redistributed her diet to provide the carbohydrate and protein coverage that she needed in the afternoon. She cheerfully complied — and hasn't had midafternoon insulin reactions since.

In another case, George, a 27-year-old lawyer, consulted us for help planning his diets for camping trips. He liked backpacking and mountain climbing on weekends, but often experienced hypoglycemic symptoms in the afternoon. We explained that exercise tends to lower blood glucose levels and usually requires altering insulin, diet, or both. Since George managed his day-to-day 2,800-calorie diet (with 3 p.m. snack) well, our only recommendation was to increase his 3 p.m. snack during backpacking trips. In a few weeks, he returned complaining that the increased calories made him feel so full that he felt uncomfortable — and he still experienced hypoglycemic reactions in the afternoon. Our next suggestion: reduce his insulin from 30 units of NPH to 20 units on the days he would be backpacking. He found that this adjustment, plus concentrated camp foods, solved his problem.

Both of these cases involved only minor compromises to solve medical problems. But sometimes you have to make major compromises simply to get a patient to adhere to a consistent diet. Insisting on an "ideal" diet with recalcitrant patients would be a waste of their time — and yours. Often, for instance, you must compromise on what you consider an adequate breakfast to get a patient to eat any breakfast at all. Or you must settle for a higher-than-recommended caloric intake to keep the patient on a consistent diet.

Oscar, for example, was far overweight at 310 lb. So, our first diet plan included a hefty reduction in calories. As we outlined the plan to Oscar, we mentioned a daily sandwich, which is what he had told us he ate every lunch. Oscar balked.

"One sandwich? That's all for lunch — every blessed day? I'll starve to death. Some days I need two sandwiches."

We started to explain the desirability of weight loss but didn't get far. Clearly we were losing him. We backed down and worked for something positive — consistency. To ensure that his caloric intake would be the same every day, we added another sandwich at every day's lunch. But we insisted that he eat two sandwiches every day. Oscar agreed. He still has his large dimensions, but at least he maintains some semblance of diabetic control.

True, this method isn't ideal. And we don't claim to have solved the ongoing dilemma of getting diabetic patients to comply with their diets. But we've learned to approach dietary planning more positively and more realistically. And we're finding that that approach usually gets positive results with the initial diet. Of course, whether dietary controls must be supplemented with oral hypoglycemic agents or insulin depends on the patient's overall condition and the severity of his diabetes.

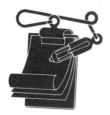

Remember these important points about enforcing dietary restrictions for diabetic patients:
1. Plan dietary programs to maintain ideal weight and proper nutrition, to assist in controlling diabetes, and to assist in preventing and controlling short-term and long-term complications.
2. Tailor your patient's diet to his life-style, considering the kind, amount, and usual time of his activity; his illnesses or other stresses; and the type of insulin he takes and his body's response to it.
3. Understand that your patient may deviate from his diet since breaking lifelong habits is difficult.
4. Forestall hypoglycemia by suggesting slower acting starches for afternoon or evening snacks.
5. Administer fast-acting sugars to treat insulin shock.

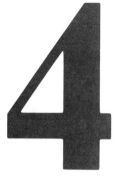

Oral agents:
When diet alone fails

BY LARRY N. GEVER, RPh, PharmD

FOR THE CHILD WHO DEVELOPS diabetes mellitus, diet and insulin are the only means of therapy. But for the Type II diabetic patient, there are two other alternatives: diet alone or diet and oral hypoglycemic agents.

The advantage of oral therapy over insulin therapy is obvious — convenience. But convenience can also be the main disadvantage. Because without the daily inconvenience of an insulin injection, some patients underrate the gravity of their diabetes and slip off their prescribed diet and medication.

For just that reason, your role in oral therapy for diabetic patients isn't as limited as you might think. Many doctors who prescribe a hypoglycemic drug tell the patient to take it once or twice a day and then send him out to manage his own therapy as best he can. In your contact with the patient, you have a tremendous opportunity to fill in what the doctor leaves out — explanations of how the drugs work, the risks, and how to keep those risks to a minimum.

Oral therapy isn't for everyone
For some diabetic patients, oral agents — the sulfonylureas, such as Orinase, for example — definitely have a place in treatment. They can't substitute for dietary controls. But as

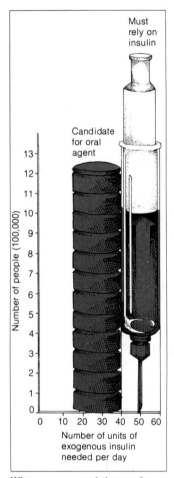

Must rely on insulin

Candidate for oral agent

Number of people (100,000)

13
12
11
10
9
8
7
6
5
4
3
2
1
0

0   10   20   30   40   50   60

Number of units of exogenous insulin needed per day

Who can use oral therapy?
The candidate for oral therapy is the nonketotic Type II diabetic patient. Control of diet and exercise is just as important as with insulin-dependent patients, perhaps more so since the convenience of oral therapy may cause the Type II diabetic patient to underestimate his condition.

adjuncts to diet and as replacements for insulin injections, they do benefit many patients both medically and psychologically. Unfortunately, though, not all Type II diabetic patients are eligible for oral therapy.

Of all the criteria doctors use to select candidates, the most critical is pancreatic function.

The normal adult pancreas secretes 40 to 60 units of insulin each day, an amount that is essential for acceptable carbohydrate metabolism.

In diabetes mellitus, the pancreas secretes too little insulin. If a diabetic patient has no pancreatic function, he needs injections of 40 to 60 units of exogenous insulin each day to prevent hyperglycemia. If he has residual pancreatic function, however, he may be able to control his condition with dietary modifications and oral agents, since the oral agents regulate blood glucose levels using endogenous insulin. A good candidate for trial on oral hypoglycemics is a patient who would require less than 40 units of exogenous insulin per day, indicating some degree of pancreatic function.

Testing pancreatic function generally rules out oral therapy for children with Type I diabetes since they characteristically have no residual pancreatic function. Without pancreatic function, they're prone to life-threatening ketoacidosis as well as hyperglycemia. These patients need complete insulin replacement.

Patients with Type II diabetes, on the other hand, often have enough pancreatic function to produce some insulin and to resist ketoacidosis. They may be able to rely on oral hypoglycemic agents to regulate their blood glucose levels.

When we draw a profile of a likely candidate for oral therapy, we find that he has diabetes mellitus, is usually over 40 years old, is ketoacidosis-resistant, can't control his condition with diet alone, and needs less than 40 units of insulin per day. Of course, some other conditions, such as pregnancy or surgery, preclude oral therapy. The candidate must meet those criteria as well.

Even if the patient does meet all the criteria for oral therapy, though, the doctor may place him on insulin. Why? Because the patient or his doctor may decide that the risks of oral therapy outweigh its advantages. For example, a major study has implicated the oral hypoglycemics in a high incidence of cardiovascular deaths among all diabetic patients, regardless of preexisting cardiovascular disease.

But if the doctor does decide to try oral therapy, he must then make another decision: which sulfonylurea to prescribe.

The "undercover" agents

Many patients mistakenly believe that hypoglycemic agents are oral insulin. Nothing could be further from the truth; there is no such thing as oral insulin. If taken orally, insulin would be degraded and have no effect. Oral hypoglycemic agents are simply synthetic agents that help reduce the blood glucose level. Exactly how they regulate the blood glucose level, though, is a matter for speculation.

Sulfonylureas seem to act primarily on the beta cells of the islets of Langerhans in the pancreas. These cells normally produce and secrete enough insulin to maintain the correct blood glucose level. As a person ages, though, these cells may become sluggish, impairing the body's response to rising blood glucose. Sulfonylureas initially stimulate the beta cells to release more insulin, thus lowering the blood glucose level.

After prolonged use, the sulfonylureas no longer cause an increase in insulin release. For some reason, however, the improvement in glucose tolerance is maintained. No one knows exactly why the sulfonylureas continue to work, but experiments suggest that the drugs may also increase glucose uptake in the peripheral tissues, resulting in decreased blood glucose levels.

A secondary function of the sulfonylureas involves the release of glucose from the liver. Normally, the liver and pancreas interact to maintain the blood glucose level. The liver stores glucose in the form of glycogen, which it reconverts to glucose and releases into the blood when needed to maintain the correct blood glucose level. To prevent the blood glucose level from rising too high, the pancreas normally releases insulin. But in a diabetic patient, the pancreas can't release enough insulin to prevent hyperglycemia from the hepatic glucose release. By inhibiting the release of hepatic glucose, the sulfonylureas help balance the deficiency in pancreatic response.

Glyburide and glipizide are the so-called second-generation sulfonylureas that:

• have greater milligram-per-milligram potency than first-generation drugs.

• are almost always prescribed on a once-daily basis. First-generation sulfonylureas (except chlorpropamide) often must

Barriers to oral therapy

• *Pregnancy.* In addition to possibly causing teratogenic effects or congenital malformations in the fetus, oral agents may not control diabetes complicated by pregnancy. Furthermore, oral agents can cross the placental barrier, inducing hypoglycemia in the neonate; insulin can't.

• *Severe stress, surgery, fever, or infection.* Any traumatic condition can trigger wide fluctuations in the patient's diabetic state, almost always demanding a temporary return to insulin therapy. Elderly patients are particularly prone to changes in response to their oral hypoglycemic agents, since their hepatic and renal functions may change markedly during illness.

• *Suspected sulfa allergy.* Any previous allergic reaction to a sulfa drug bars sulfonylurea therapy, since the sulfonylureas are chemically related to the sulfonamide antimicrobial category of drugs.

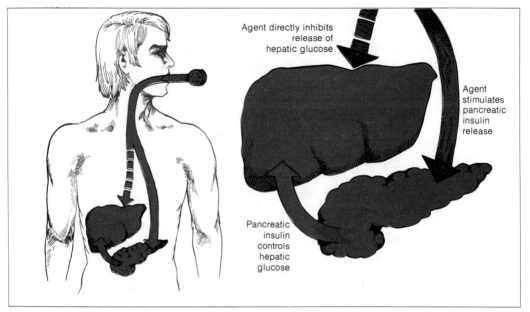

Agent directly inhibits release of hepatic glucose

Agent stimulates pancreatic insulin release

Pancreatic insulin controls hepatic glucose

How do sulfonylureas work?
To be effective, sulfonylureas require either insulin-producing beta cells or the presence of some exogenous insulin. In receptive individuals they increase the manufacture and release of insulin in response to food and increase the glucose uptake in fat and in muscle. They may or may not decrease the secretion of glucagon, a pancreatic hormone that raises blood glucose levels. Under certain circumstances sulfonylureas may stimulate the formation of new beta cells.

be prescribed on a twice-daily basis.

• are inactivated by the liver and so are safer than chlorpropamide in patients with renal insufficiency.

• have side effects generally similar to those of the first-generation drugs. However, the disulfiram-like reaction seen with first-generation drugs is rare with glyburide and glipizide.

• may provide good control for patients who've experienced failure with first-generation sulfonylureas.

• carry the same risk of increased cardiovascular mortality as the first-generation drugs.

• are prescribed in dosages 2.5 to 5 mg once daily (glyburide) or 5 mg once daily (glipizide).

However the oral agents achieve their effects, all have a single goal: to regulate the blood glucose level. Naturally, though, the oral hypoglycemics do vary in duration of action, dosages, and metabolism (see table opposite). These elements influence the doctor's choice of an oral hypoglycemic agent for a particular patient.

Chlorpropamide (Diabinese), which is excreted unchanged in the urine, is the longest-acting oral agent. Since its effect may last as long as 36 hours, a patient usually has to take it only once a day.

Tolazamide (Tolinase) and *acetohexamide (Dymelor)* are intermediate agents that are metabolized in the liver. In fact, acetohexamide *must* be metabolized to be an active drug.

Comparison of Oral Hypoglycemics

GENERIC NAME	TRADE NAME	DOSAGE FORM	USUAL DAILY DOSE	DURATION OF ACTION
tolbutamide	Orinase	500 mg	1 to 2 g daily as single dose or in divided doses b.i.d. or t.i.d.	6 to 12 hr
tolazamide	Tolinase	100 mg 250 mg	100 to 500 mg as single dose or in divided doses b.i.d. with breakfast and supper	12 to 24 hr
acetohexamide	Dymelor	250 mg 500 mg	250 mg daily up to 1.5 g in divided doses b.i.d. to t.i.d. before meals	12 to 24 hr
chlorpropamide	Diabinese	100 mg 250 mg	250 to 750 mg daily as single dose or in divided doses if GI disturbance occurs	24 to 36 hr
glipizide	Glucotrol	5 mg 10 mg	5 mg daily as single dose	24 hr
glyburide	Diabeta, Micronase	1.25 mg 2.5 mg 5 mg	2.5 to 5 mg daily as single dose	24 hr

The patient may be able to rely on once-a-day therapy with acetohexamide or tolazamide, although two daily doses may be necessary.

Tolbutamide (Orinase), also metabolized in the liver, is the most rapid-acting sulfonylurea. It must be taken two or three times a day to achieve a maximal effect.

From this information, you can see that, for once-a-day convenience, chlorpropamide would be the drug of choice. Obviously, though, convenience isn't the only criterion for selection.

For example, one drawback of chlorpropamide is that it poses a greater risk of hypoglycemia since it is so long-acting. On the other hand, with rapid-acting agents, patients often forget to take the prescribed number of doses each day.

Preexisting renal or hepatic damage also plays an important role in the selection of the correct hypoglycemic. For example, it would be unwise to treat a diabetic patient with severe liver disease with any sulfonylurea other than chlorpropamide. All the other sulfonylureas undergo liver metabolism. (Acetohexamide must be metabolized to be active. Tolbutamide and tolazamide are metabolized to less active compounds for excretion; a decrease in liver metabolism could result in toxicity from either drug.) By the same

Canadian equivalents
In Canada, some names of oral hypoglycemic agents, particularly trade names, differ from the U.S. names. Here's a Canadian listing with the usual daily maintenance doses for each:
- *acetohexamide:* Dimelor (250 mg to 1.5 g)
- *chlorpropamide:* Chloromide, Chloronase, Diabinese, Novopropamide, Stabinol (100 to 500 mg)
- *glyburide:* Euglucon, Diabeta (2.5 to 20 mg)
- *tolbutamide:* Mellitol, Mobenol, Neo-Dibetic, Novobutamide, Oramide, Orinase, Tolbutone (0.5 to 3 g)

One a day

For the Type II diabetic patient whose diabetes is well controlled, remembering to take his daily dose of medication may be his biggest problem.

To help this patient keep track of his medication, the manufacturer of chlorpropramide (Diabinese) has developed this new packaging. It takes advantage of the same packaging concept that birth control pills use to supply a month's supply of medication. If the patient can afford this more expensive packaging, he will be able to tell at a glance whether or not he's taken his daily dose.

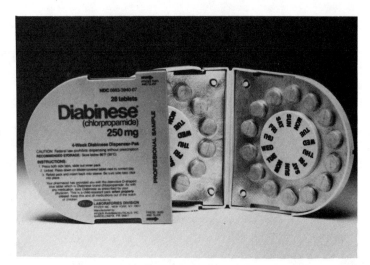

token, caution should be taken with a diabetic patient with renal insufficiency using chlorpropramide or acetohexamide, since those drugs are excreted by the kidneys in an active form. Decreased kidney function would cause them to accumulate in the blood, leading to possible toxicity.

The choice of drug, however, is the doctor's responsibility. Yours is to make sure the patient understands the hows and whys of oral therapy, the pitfalls as well as the benefits.

Hard facts and caveats

Because they don't have to take an insulin injection every day, many patients on oral therapy tend to underrate the seriousness of their diabetes and the importance of treatment.

But the cold facts are that patients on oral therapy face risks and complications just as insulin-dependent diabetic patients do. You must make a concerted effort to teach patients on oral therapy about dietary and drug management and about possible side effects.

For the patient on oral therapy, as for the insulin-dependent patient, the word *diet* goes hand in hand with diabetes. Indeed, for a patient on oral agents who is relying on his endogenous insulin supply, diet plays a particularly crucial role.

The doctor will prescribe the patient's individual diet, selecting it according to his age, ideal weight, medical condition, activity, and eating habits. For the patient with diabetes mellitus, the doctor will choose a diet from the American Diabetes

Association list (see Appendices), with a balanced level of carbohydrate, protein, and fat intake.

Whatever the diet selected for a particular patient, you should reinforce the doctor's and dietitian's instructions, explaining the need for the balanced ratio of protein, carbohydrates, and fat. Be sure, too, to emphasize the ''no cheating'' rule, that effective therapy is based on the patient eating all prescribed foods. A rule of thumb for all diabetic patients: undereating is just as hazardous as overeating.

Remind the patient that he may have to reduce his medication intake if he has a change in his level of physical activity, but that he should do so only with his doctor's approval. No self-prescribing.

To monitor the effects of diet, exercise, and medications on blood glucose levels, some doctors have their patients perform periodic urine tests, particularly during their first few weeks on therapy. Teaching them how to perform these tests will probably be your job. (See Chapters 6 and 7 for teaching instructions.) If the patient consistently gets very high or very low results, he should report them to his doctor. The doctor then may amend his dosage instructions, change the patient to another oral hypoglycemic agent, or, in persistently severe cases, change the patient to insulin.

After the patient has been on oral therapy for a while and is well controlled, he may not have to test his urine except when he suspects adverse reactions.

You also should instruct patients on oral hypoglycemic therapy about foot care. Just like the insulin-dependent patient, the oral therapy patient is susceptible to foot infections and diabetic gangrene. Show him how to care for his feet just as you would show a patient on insulin (see Chapter 6).

After you've given these initial instructions to your patient, make sure he has understood them. Question him, or reverse roles and have him explain urine tests, diet, and foot care to you. Even after you're sure he understands the instructions, follow up with periodic pep talks if possible.

Perhaps the most helpful information you can give a diabetic patient on oral therapy is how to get the best mileage out of his medication with the least risk. The key is timing, both in the number of doses per day and the time of administration.

Frequency of administration depends on the particular agent, the patient's medical condition, and his response to therapy.

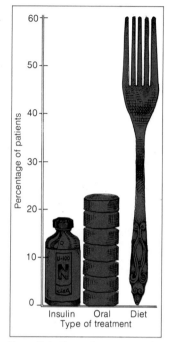

How diabetic patients control their condition
Many diabetic patients are able to control their condition by diet alone, an encouraging fact. Other patients combine methods, however, watching what they eat *and* taking insulin or oral hypoglycemics. Combinations are not represented in the above chart.

Oral hypoglycemics aren't for everyone
Thin Type II diabetic patients have responded less well to oral treatment than have overweight patients. In those who do respond well, however, blood glucose levels are more nearly normal than would be possible with insulin.

Generally, the longest-acting agent, chlorpropamide, should be taken only once a day, in the morning. Drugs with shorter durations of action, such as tolbutamide, may be taken as often as two or three times a day. Find out the doctor's instructions and reinforce them.

Also impress your patient with two caveats of drug therapy.

First, if he is fasting for any reason — impending surgery or laboratory studies — he shouldn't take oral agents. Taking oral agents during fasting risks hypoglycemic reactions, since the glucose intake is decreased. In addition, the stress caused by the surgery or tests may cause fluctuations in the diabetic state, which may not be well controlled with the oral agents.

Second, he should not take his oral hypoglycemic at bedtime unless he has a special order from his attending doctor, since he could have a severe hypoglycemic reaction in his sleep. If you're caring for a diabetic patient on oral therapy in the hospital, don't give the oral agent at bedtime unless you're sure the order is valid. Have the order verified and notify your supervisor before giving the dose.

A rundown of risks
Both of these caveats underline an important point about oral therapy: oral hypoglycemic agents are potent drugs, possibly even suicidal weapons, that must be treated with the same respect accorded to insulin. The sulfonylureas can produce dangerous side effects and adverse reactions. In a study conducted by the University Group Diabetes Program, diabetic patients treated for 5 to 8 years with diet plus a fixed dose of tolbutamide (1.5 g/day) had a cardiovascular mortality two and one half times that of patients treated with diet alone. Interestingly, other studies have not confirmed these results.

Naturally, you don't want to frighten your patient by over-emphasizing the risks of oral therapy. Although he should be warned of the potential risks, you want to emphasize the positive so that he follows dietary precautions and handles his medication carefully. So, realistically explain adverse reactions; make sure your patient can recognize them in their incipient stages and can correct them swiftly. Also emphasize, though, that the risks are almost nil *if* he scrupulously follows his doctor's orders.

• *Hypoglycemia*. The greatest threat in sulfonylurea therapy is hypoglycemia, which curiously is the drug's therapeutic effect taken to extremes. Although hypoglycemia occurs infrequently with the sulfonylureas, it can cause severe illness, coma, or even death if it goes unrecognized and uncorrected.

Hypoglycemia can be precipitated by several conditions: changes in renal or hepatic function, fever, infection, surgery, or other stressful situations. For that reason, instruct your patient to call his doctor promptly at the first signs of illness. In cases of trauma or illness, the doctor may switch him temporarily to insulin therapy, since the insulin allows more individualized treatment.

Hypoglycemic effects of the sulfonylureas are potentiated by many drugs, including propranolol (Inderal) and other beta-adrenergic blockers, probenecid (Benemid), phenylbutazone (Azolid, Butazolidin), chloramphenicol (Chloromycetin), dicumarol (Dicumarol), clofibrate (Atromid-S), sulfonamide-type antibacterial agents, and high doses of salicylates. Since aspirin can lower the blood glucose level, be sure patients know to take Tylenol instead. Overdosage of oral hypoglycemics and undereating may also predispose a patient to hypoglycemia. List for the patient the early signs of hypoglycemic reactions: lethargy, sweating, hunger, inability to concentrate, shakiness, slight nervousness, irritability, dizziness, headaches, palpitations, or tremors.

If a patient experiences any of these mild reactions, he can stem them quickly by simply eating any glucose-producing food — fruit juice, soft drinks, or candy. (See Chapter 11 for details on ways to stem hypoglycemia.) If his symptoms don't subside within 10 to 15 minutes, he should take another dose of candy or soft drinks and, if possible, test his urine. If symptoms still persist after 10 or 15 minutes and his urine proves negative, he should call his doctor.

Although severe hypoglycemic reactions rarely occur with oral therapy, they can develop if mild reactions go untreated for a long period. Severe hypoglycemic reactions are characterized by grogginess, stupor, and unconsciousness. If the patient is simply groggy, a family member should place some cake-decorating frosting (the kind that comes in tubes) along his gumline and cheek. His mucous membranes will absorb the substance, and the patient should revive enough to drink a glass of fruit juice. If the patient becomes unconscious, however, he should be taken to a hospital emergency room, where he'll probably require I.V. glucose.

Phenformin: Available for those few who still need it

Phenformin (formerly DBI-TD), a biguanide oral hypoglycemic agent, was removed from the U.S. market in 1977 because its use became associated with an unacceptably high risk of lactic acidosis.

A select group of patients require phenformin to control their diabetes mellitus, however. Recognizing this, the Food and Drug Administration (FDA) has made the drug available through an Investigational New Drug (IND) application, which a prescribing doctor must file with the FDA.

According to the FDA, phenformin may be used only in non-ketotic diabetic patients who meet *all* the following criteria:
• elevated blood glucose levels
• signs and symptoms, such as polydipsia
• lack of control of signs and symptoms by diet or sulfonylureas (or hypersensitivity to sulfonylurea)
• evidence that phenformin controls the patient's signs and symptoms
• no underlying risk factors that contraindicate use of phenformin
• risk of hypoglycemia from insulin, threatening the patient's job or posing a hazard to him or others
• disability, if the disability makes the patient unable to take insulin without help and he has no practical way to get the help he needs.

If your patient's taking phenformin, make sure he understands the signs and symptoms that herald the onset of lactic acidosis: nausea, vomiting, hyperventilation, malaise, or abdominal pain. If any of these occur, he should stop the drug and notify his doctor immediately. Also advise your patient to avoid alcoholic beverages while taking phenformin.

Scientific serendipity
The road to the discovery of oral hypoglycemics was paved with serendipity and coincidence. In 1942, Marcel Janbon, a Frenchman, was working with sulfa drugs to treat cases of typhoid when he found that one sulfa drug derivative (IPTD) lowered the blood glucose levels of his patients to the point of producing convulsions. Janbon's colleague, Auguste Loubatieres, began a prolonged series of animal studies to identify the cause. By 1955, Loubatieres had discovered that IPTD exerted no hypoglycemic effect in pancreatectomized animals. From this he deduced that the drug stimulated the pancreas to secrete insulin.

Neither Janbon nor Loubatieres, however, explored sulfa drugs' usefulness in diabetes treatment. Instead Hans Franke and J. Fuchs, German scientists studying the hypoglycemic action of sulfa drugs, found that the antibacterial agent carbutamide lowered blood glucose levels. They demonstrated its usefulness in the treatment of diabetes, and soon after the first oral hypoglycemic was introduced.

Another treatment for hypoglycemic reaction is glucagon, a hormone produced by the alpha cells of the pancreatic islets of Langerhans. Like insulin, which is produced by the beta cells, glucagon is derived from animals. When administered to a patient, this extracted hormone raises blood glucose levels by converting glycogen to glucose in the liver.

To reconstitute the glucagon powder for injection, add it to the sterile diluent provided in the package. Use *only* the diluent provided. Once it's reconstituted, glucagon may be given I.V., intramuscularly, or subcutaneously.

Administer 0.5 to 1 mg (unit) by one of these routes. Usually, the patient will respond 5 to 10 minutes later. If he doesn't, you may give one or two more doses. If he doesn't respond after 20 minutes, administer 50 to 100 ml of I.V. 50% dextrose to prevent cerebral hypoglycemia — a life-threatening condition.

When the patient does respond, give him oral carbohydrates followed by a protein snack. This is necessary because the glucose produced by glucagon quickly goes back into the cells, and the patient again risks hypoglycemia.

Monitor his vital signs, level of consciousness, and blood glucose levels every 2 hours for 24 hours. Encourage him to rest, since hypoglycemia is extremely stressful. When he's recovered, review with him how to avoid hypoglycemia.

If the patient is subject to frequent hypoglycemic reactions, teach his family how to administer glucagon.

• *Change in level of consciousness.* Any marked change in consciousness indicates the need for rapid medical attention. The correct diagnosis for the cause of the change is essential.

• *Hyperglycemia.* Naturally if a patient forgets to take his medication regularly, he can have a return of his initial symptoms of hyperglycemia. And he may be more prone to hyperglycemia if he is taking thiazide diuretics, which aggravate the diabetic state and may increase requirements for oral agents. (Other drugs may also cause hyperglycemia. Rifampin, for example, may increase an oral hypoglycemic's metabolic breakdown, thus making the drug less effective.) Symptoms of hyperglycemia, usually vague and mild at first, include loss of appetite, lethargy, nausea, vomiting, a high urine glucose level, a positive urine acetone reading, frequent urination, and marked thirst. If untreated for a prolonged period, the patient's condition could worsen and eventually progress to diabetic coma.

The best way to ward off hyperglycemia, of course, is to follow dietary and drug instructions. A patient with mild symptoms usually can correct them by returning to his prescribed regimen. For persistent, severe symptoms, however, the patient should be seen by his doctor; he may require insulin and fluid replacement therapy to correct the hyperglycemia.

• *Alcohol intolerance and other adverse reactions.* One side effect of the sulfonylureas, especially chlorpropamide (Diabinese), is an disulfiram-like reaction, which may occur when a patient drinks alcoholic beverages. In fact, the patient may appear drunk — stumbling, slurring his words, having trouble remembering. He also may be flushed, nauseated, and tachycardic. Although alcohol intolerance usually is mild, it can cause severe headaches and vomiting and can produce symptoms lasting up to 1 hour.

The best cure for this reaction is the avoidance of alcohol. Warn your patient to be careful when he drinks. If he experiences any symptoms of alcohol intolerance, he should eliminate his drinking.

Just for reference, you also should know that the sulfonylureas alone can produce a host of side effects: anorexia, nausea, vomiting, diarrhea, blood dyscrasias, hemolytic anemia, and allergic skin reactions (usually transient). Gastrointestinal irritation is the most common side effect and may call for a reduction in dose or the use of divided drug therapy.

Serious side effects are rare, but they should be reported immediately to the doctor. Sometimes the side effects can be easily corrected by adjusting the dosage or by switching to another hypoglycemic agent or insulin.

A patient on oral therapy may complain of headaches and weakness a couple of hours after eating. These symptoms could mean that the patient needs a smaller dose of his drug or that his diet is not balanced. If he complains of these symptoms, have him record his food intake. You may be able to eliminate the symptoms simply by adjusting his diet or urging him to stick to it more closely. If the symptoms persist, report them to the doctor.

Two different outcomes

How well does oral therapy work for patients? Should you take particular precautions with particular patients? Is oral

Some Actions of Insulin and Sulfonylureas		
	INSULIN	SULFONYLUREAS
Major action	• Increased glucose transfer into cells	• Increased insulin secretion
Subsidiary effects: • Insulin secretion	• Decreased	• Increased
• Glucose uptake by peripheral tissues	• Increased	• Increased
• Blood glucose–lowering effect: —Normal subjects —Depancreatized subjects	• Marked • Marked	• Moderate • None
• Marked hypoglycemia • Lactate utilization • Irreversible side effects	• Common • Increased • Present	• Rare • Increased • Rare

therapy always successful? The following examples may help answer those questions.

Mildred, a wiry 40 year old, had an almost classic case of Type II diabetes mellitus, discovered in an almost classic way. For several months she had seemed a different person, snapping at her colleagues at work for no apparent reason and feeling constantly irritable. Her concentration also slipped; she often broke into tears at the slightest provocation; and she constantly felt exhausted, thirsty, and hungry. Even though she snacked every couple of hours, her hunger and thirst persisted and she also began losing weight.

For a while, she accepted the opinion of sympathetic friends who said it was "change of life." But when she began having to struggle to keep her weight up, she finally consulted a doctor. He promptly sent her to the hospital for a workup, including a fasting blood glucose test. The test showed an abnormally high level, 160 mg/dl, so the doctor ordered a 2-hour postprandial blood glucose test, which also was elevated at 170 mg/dl.

Mildred's doctor started her on acetohexamide at a standard dose of 250 mg twice a day, before breakfast and before dinner. Within a few days, Mildred began to feel like herself again. And within a week or so she was completely rid of her insatiable hunger. In fact, she felt so good that, like many new diabetic patients, she often forgot to take her pills.

When Mildred returned to the doctor's office complaining again of her earlier symptoms, the nurse explained diabetes to her. She emphasized that oral therapy is not a cure but rather a way to avert serious problems now and in the future. But, she said, it could be effective only if Mildred followed the prescribed regimen to the letter. She showed her how to keep a chart of her daily medications. And she stressed that her role was simply that of an advising nurse, not a nursemaid; Mildred would have to take full custody of her own daily care.

With these explanations, Mildred was soon back on her therapy schedule. Now, more than 3 years after she began therapy, she is still successfully managing her condition with Dymelor.

Unfortunately, though, not all patients have such success. Some may not be able to take oral agents from the start (primary failure); others start off well on them and then, for some unknown reason, the drugs seem to lose their effectiveness (secondary failure). Steve, for example, discovered his diabetes when he came into the hospital for a hernia repair. Tests showed his fasting blood glucose level to be 180 mg/dl and consistently elevated levels in his glucose tolerance.

At first the doctors placed Steve on insulin therapy in the hospital, since his surgery, minor as it was, caused his diabetic state to fluctuate considerably. Just before he was discharged, though, they switched him to tolbutamide, 500 mg twice a day. Steve left the hospital. Within a week, he was back with a blood glucose level just as high as it had been before. After a long talk with him, the nurse was convinced that he had been taking his pills and hadn't been cheating on his diet. The doctor slowly increased Steve's tolbutamide dose to the recommended maximum of 3 g daily.

When Steve's diabetes was not controlled at that dose, the doctor decided that his condition just couldn't be controlled with oral therapy. He switched Steve to Lente insulin. Within a few days, Steve's condition stabilized.

No one knows why patients like Steve don't succeed on oral therapy. Some have even been able to get along on as little as 18 units of insulin a day (a dose that indicates fairly strong pancreatic functioning) but still can't rely on oral medications. Fortunately, though, these patients are the exception rather than the rule. Diabetic patients who do benefit from their oral hypoglycemic therapy, both medically and psychologically, deserve the opportunity to use that treatment You can provide them with a much needed service by remembering that they are still diabetic patients and by teaching and encouraging them accordingly.

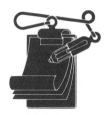

Remember these important points about diabetic patients and oral agents:
1. Consider a patient requiring less than 40 units of exogenous insulin daily a good candidate for an oral hypoglycemic agent.
2. Be aware of oral therapy's contraindications: pregnancy, severe stress, surgery, fever or infection, suspected sulfa allergy, and a predisposition to lactic acidosis.
3. Know that sulfonylureas work by increasing the manufacture and release of insulin in response to food and by increasing the glucose uptake in fat and muscle.
4. Understand that when selecting an oral hypoglycemic agent for your patient, the doctor considers the drug's duration of action and dosage, as well as the patient's metabolism.
5. Watch for such side effects as hypoglycemia, change in level of consciousness, hyperglycemia, and alcohol intolerance.

5

Insulin:
Easing the daily routine

BY LAWRENCE W. WOLFE, BSC, RPH

JUST BECAUSE insulin therapy becomes a daily routine for some diabetic patients, don't think it's simple. Even nurses in hospitals make mistakes in insulin therapy — mismatching concentrations and syringes, confusing the different types of insulin, ignoring the best injection time for rapid-acting and long-acting insulins, even neglecting to rotate injection sites.

You could hardly call it child's play. Yet it's life-saving therapy for about 500,000 to 600,000 Type I, or insulin-dependent, diabetic patients. Ironically, about half are under age 19. As with oral or dietary therapy, you'll probably be the person responsible for teaching patients both the practices and pitfalls of this therapy. You must know how insulin works and how insulin therapy can be adapted to each patient's needs.

Just what is insulin?
As explained in Chapter 1, insulin is a major anabolic hormone that regulates the body's carbohydrate, fat, and protein metabolism. It acts primarily in the liver, adipose tissue, and muscle to promote glucose uptake, stimulate glycogen synthesis, and suppress glucose production. When a patient's body fails to produce enough insulin or the insulin produced isn't used correctly, the patient has to control his glucose

Types of Insulin				
INSULIN	ONSET	PEAK	DURATION	APPEARANCE
Rapid-acting				
Regular	30 to 60 min	3 to 5 hr	5 to 8 hr	Clear
Semilente	30 to 60 min	4 to 6 hr	12 to 16 hr	Cloudy
Intermediate				
NPH	60 to 90 min	8 to 12 hr	24 to 28 hr	Cloudy
Lente	60 to 90 min	8 to 12 hr	24 to 28 hr	Cloudy
Long-acting				
PZI	3 to 6 hr	14 to 20 hr	36 + hr	Cloudy
Ultralente	5 to 8 hr	16 to 18 hr	36 + hr	Cloudy

Canadian equivalents
Generally, names of the various insulins are the same in Canada as in the United States. However, Canada has a Sulfated insulin for insulin-resistant diabetic patients who need more than 200 units daily. (With Sulfated insulin, these patients can manage their diabetes on one tenth to one fifth their previous dose.) Also, U-500 isn't available in Canada.

intake through diet and may have to either stimulate insulin production with oral agents or supplement his endogenous insulin with injections of exogenous (beef or pork) insulin.

Unfortunately, many nurses fail to explain the variations in the types of insulin when they teach insulin therapy to new diabetic patients. Perhaps they assume that patients would only become confused by an "information overload" about medications they won't be taking. On the contrary, I have found that many patients become confused by a *lack* of information. Without understanding the variables in insulin therapy, they may use the wrong syringe with their insulin, mistime their injections, or skip doses.

There are, of course, several types of insulin. These fall into three general categories: rapid-acting (quick uptake and short duration — regular and Semilente), intermediate (NPH and Lente), and long-acting (slow uptake and long duration — PZI and Ultralente).

Within these categories, each type of insulin has its own onset, peak, and duration of action (see chart above). The variety in action, coupled with varieties in concentrations and doses, allows a doctor to tailor insulin therapy to each patient's highly individual needs. (You'll notice that NPH and Lente have about the same onset and duration of action. However, they differ in basic makeup. NPH insulin contains zinc and two proteins — protamine and globin — to prolong its action. By utilizing 10 times more zinc, Lente — composed of Semilente and Ultralente — achieves the same duration without any foreign modifying protein. So it can be used by patients who are allergic to the proteins in NPH).

In nearly all hospitals, U-100 insulin is the preferred concentration replacing U-40. (U-80 insulin is no longer available.) The term U-100 refers to the concentration of insulin per milliliter of liquid — in this case, 100 units/ml. U-100 concentration should be used only with a U-100 syringe (a syringe calibrated in 100 units). In hospitals that don't use U-100 insulin exclusively, one of the leading causes of dosage errors is mismatching the syringe and concentration.

You can easily see how such a dosage error can occur. If a patient requires 20 units of U-100 insulin and it's administered in a U-40 syringe, the dosage will be more than twice the prescribed amount. In another example, if the patient requires 20 units of U-40 insulin and it's administered in a U-100 syringe, the dosage will be less than half the prescribed amount.

All U-100 insulin today is "single-peak" — a highly purified product containing approximately 90% insulin and 9% insulin-like substances. Older products contained only 92% of these components and caused far more antigenicity.

Single component insulin (human or pork), which is 99% pure insulin, is prescribed when a patient has:
• an insulin allergy (local cutaneous reaction)
• an insulin resistance (more than 100 units required per day)
• lipoatrophy or lipohypertrophy
• type II diabetes mellitus requiring short-term insulin use (such as during pregnancy, surgery, or intravenous hyperalimentation).

U-500 insulin also is available for treatment of coma and cases of insulin resistance requiring large doses of insulin.

The chart on page 50 summarizes the onset, peak, and duration of each type of insulin based on the average person's response. But not all patients are average. Some may respond differently, depending on several conditions:
• *Route of administration.* Most insulins must be given subcutaneously; only regular insulin may be given intravenously. Insulin can be given intramuscularly for a faster onset in emergencies, but the onset with I.M. administration can be unpredictable, so most doctors prefer I.V. administration.
• *Vascularity of the injection site.* Commonly used injection sites, such as the upper arms, thighs, and stomach, have a high degree of vascularity, which prompts absorption of insulin. Absorption will slow if the patient's vascular system is impaired — for example, from muscular atrophy, edema, renal disease, or some systemic diseases.
• *Physical changes in the insulin.* These include chemical

Human insulin:
Some pros and cons
Although most insulin comes from pork or beef, human insulin — as the name implies — is derived from a recombined form of the DNA molecule. Scientists had hoped insulin from a human source would eliminate the risk of allergic reactions, but this isn't so. In fact, the incidence of allergic reactions with human insulin is nearly identical to that of highly purified (monocomponent) pork insulin: low but not zero. Some experts suggest that these reactions are caused not by the insulin itself but by the subcutaneous injection of insulin molecules and noninsulin protein contained in the solution.

Currently, human insulin is available in regular and NPH forms. Human insulin's onset and duration is shorter than beef- or pork-based products, which means it has to be injected more frequently. In most markets, human insulin is priced competitively with pure pork insulin.

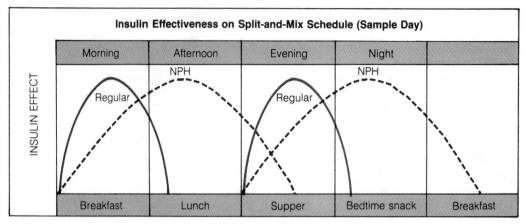

Insulin Effectiveness on Split-and-Mix Schedule (Sample Day)

Morning	Afternoon	Evening	Night	
Breakfast	Lunch	Supper	Bedtime snack	Breakfast

INSULIN EFFECT

Regular — NPH — Regular — NPH

Split-and-mix schedule
Some doctors may prefer a split-and-mix dosing schedule — that is, the patient divides and alternates regular and modified insulin doses throughout the day. A split-and-mix schedule provides the patient with enough insulin for every meal as well as for overnight. Depending on the patient's routine food intake and activity level, the split-and-mix dosing schedule has four common variations:
• regular-NPH insulin (or Lente) before breakfast and again before supper (two injections)
• regular-NPH insulin (or Lente) before breakfast, regular insulin before supper, and NPH insulin (Lente) at bedtime (three injections)
• regular insulin before each meal and NPH insulin (Lente) at bedtime (four injections)
• regular insulin and long-acting insulin (PZI or Ultralente) at breakfast; regular insulin at each subsequent meal (three injections).
Whatever the variation, be sure the patient understands that he must adhere to his basic meal plan and activity level to avoid skewing his dose. If he deviates from his meal plan, he must proportionately adjust his insulin dosage or activity level.

deterioration and contamination by other types of insulin.
• *Concentration.* As concentration increases, so does the duration of the insulin effect.
• *Biological and physiologic variations.* Different patients may respond differently to the same dose of insulin.
Patients should know that any of the above conditions could affect their response to insulin and that they should contact their doctor for a change in dose.

Timing, storing, and mixing
Just as important as getting the right insulin in the right dose is taking it at the right time. Patients don't need an intricate timetable for each individual type of insulin, but they should understand the rationale for timing doses.
Generally, patients on rapid-acting insulin should take it about 30 minutes before meals. Since it begins working within 20 to 45 minutes, this timing will ensure enough glucose intake at onset to prevent hyperinsulinism. All intermediate and long-acting insulins should be taken about 1 hour before meals. That will allow a leeway for their delayed onset.
Preparation for injection really begins with storage of the insulin bottle. All insulin will remain potent up to 36 months in a refrigerator and up to 18 to 24 months at room temperature (68° to 70° F., or 20° to 21° C.). At high temperatures (around 100° F., or 37.8° C), insulin loses its potency within a couple of months; when frozen, it remains potent but the insulin may collect in tiny clumps, making withdrawal of a uniform dose difficult. Generally, though, a patient shouldn't worry about potency if he uses his common sense in storing his insulin. As long as he avoids leaving it in the glove compartment of a hot car or on the shelf during a long hot spell, the insulin

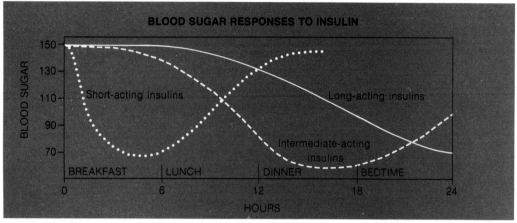

BLOOD SUGAR RESPONSES TO INSULIN

Short-acting insulins

Long-acting insulins

Intermediate-acting insulins

BREAKFAST | LUNCH | DINNER | BEDTIME

BLOOD SUGAR

HOURS

should remain stable until the expiration date marked on the label.

If a patient is unsure about the potency of a bottle of insulin, though, he can easily check it by examining its color. Regular insulin should be clear; all other types should be cloudy and free of clumps or aggregations. If they don't meet these requirements, he should discard the bottle.

Chapter 6 graphically shows the proper techniques for drawing up and injecting a single dose of insulin. If the patient must mix regular insulin with an intermediate insulin, he should first make sure both are the same concentration. Then he should follow stringent guidelines for mixing insulins. For example, if he should take 15 units of NPH and 5 units of regular insulin, he would follow this protocol:

• Observing aseptic precautions, inject 15 units of air into the bottle of NPH insulin and withdraw the needle.

• Inject 5 units of air into the regular insulin bottle and withdraw 5 units of insulin. Eliminate all air bubbles from the barrel of the syringe and the hub of the needle.

• Insert the needle into the bottle of NPH insulin, making sure the needle doesn't rest in the air space above the fluid. Withdraw 15 units of NPH insulin. (By injecting 15 units of air into the NPH insulin bottle during the first step, the patient creates positive pressure within the bottle. This prevents the regular insulin in the syringe from leaking into the bottle and contaminating the NPH insulin.)

Insulin infusion pump as an option
If you're caring for a Type I, or insulin-dependent, diabetic patient who has erratic blood glucose levels despite following a prescribed regimen, an insulin infusion pump may be the

Peaks vary
You can see why doctors prescribe insulin with different lengths of action. They keep the patient's blood glucose level well within normal limits because they peak at different times.

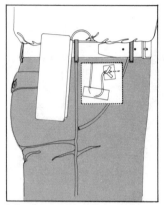

Infusion pumps: Two choices
Insulin infusion pumps — both the closed-loop and open-loop units — satisfy a diabetic patient's special insulin needs.

The *closed-loop* (self-contained) system can sense and react to changes in blood glucose levels. Unfortunately, the only commercially available system — Biostator Glucose Controller — is very large ($18'' \times 7'' \times 5''$), and requires an I.V. line to withdraw blood and infuse insulin. You'll rarely find it outside a hospital. It's usually used to meet the insulin needs of diabetic patients undergoing surgery or of those in a ketoacidotic state, in labor or delivery, or in need of an insulin adjustment. While attached to this controller, the patient can eat his usual meals and snacks and exercise by riding a stationary bicycle or walking on a treadmill.

The *open-loop* system, also known as the continuous subcutaneous insulin infusion (CSII) pump, automatically delivers insulin in small (basal) doses every few minutes and manually infuses large (bolus) doses on demand. About half the daily insulin dosage is given in basal doses; the other half in boluses. However, the open-loop system *(continued on next page)*

answer. This small electromechanical device helps control a patient's blood glucose level by automatically infusing a regular basal dose of insulin, allowing him to manually infuse larger doses before meals or intense physical activity. Also, the patient avoids the discomfort of an injection with each dose.

But not all diabetic patients are candidates for infusion pump therapy. An acceptable candidate must:
• have consistently erratic blood glucose levels and be receiving at least three injections of rapid-acting or intermediate insulin daily
• be following his prescribed diabetes regimen and be knowledgeable about his care
• have been monitoring his own blood glucose levels four times daily for at least 2 months
• be pregnant or planning a pregnancy and be willing to monitor her blood glucose levels four times a day, follow a prescribed regimen, and be knowledgeable about diabetes care.

No matter how carefully a doctor calculates a patient's insulin dose, chances are he'll have to modify it periodically to adapt to changes in the patient's health and life-style. Each patient should check his urine or blood glucose regularly, as he would with oral hypoglycemic agents, to assess his changing needs. Based on these results, the patient will make changes in his insulin dosage, according to his doctor's guidelines.

In addition to these adjustments, a patient may have to change his insulin dose during periods of extreme stress or exercise. Unless his doctor has authorized him to make dosage adjustments himself, though, he should consult his doctor before making any changes.

Hazards remain, local reactions wane
The hazards of diabetes — neuropathies, ketoacidosis, retinopathy, cardiovascular disorders, and so forth — threaten a patient on insulin as they do patients on oral hypoglycemic agents or diet alone. In fact, in some cases they threaten the insulin patient more because his condition is more severe. Still, with careful adherence to therapy, and with such daily precautions as foot care, patients can minimize the threats.

Coming chapters will thoroughly discuss the most serious systemic reactions to insulin therapy — insulin-induced shock and HHNC — as well as the ever-present threat of ketoacidosis. But there are also less serious but equally important local reactions.

Some patients, particularly young women, suffer from facial edema and sometimes edema of the extremities from insulin injections. This usually subsides within a couple of days. If not, the doctor may prescribe a low-salt diet and a mild diuretic. About 30% of all patients develop painful edema around the injection site, which also subsides within a couple of days.

Fortunately the advent of single-peak (purified) insulin has cut the incidence of these reactions. But you should forewarn patients so they don't become overly concerned if they experience them.

A small percentage of patients develop fatty atrophy at injection sites. Although dimpling usually is minor, some patients may develop craterlike cavities measuring 4″ to 5″ in diameter and up to 3″ deep. Usually, though, rotation of injection sites will prevent such serious complications.

Insulin therapy certainly isn't simple. But with the above instructions, most patients — even young children — will soon be managing it with few difficulties.

Remember these important points about insulin:
1. Know the three general insulin categories: rapid-acting, intermediate, and long-acting.
2. Be alert for conditions affecting patient response, such as administration route changes, injection site vascularity, physical changes in the insulin, and physiologic variations.
3. Advise the patient using a rapid-acting insulin to take it about 30 minutes before meals; intermediate and long-acting insulin should be taken about 1 hour before meals.
4. Consider a highly motivated type I diabetic patient or a pregnant diabetic patient a candidate for an insulin infusion pump.
5. Emphasize the importance of adhering to a diet and exercise routine in maintaining consistent blood glucose levels.

Infusion pumps: Two choices
(continued)
does not respond to changes in blood glucose levels.

The open-loop pump, shown on the opposite page, is made of high-impact plastic and is powered by disposable or rechargeable batteries. Because it's small and lightweight, the pump can be worn on a belt or placed in a pocket. It consists of a syringe (to hold the insulin), a syringe holder, and a mechanism to drive the plunger. By depressing the plunger, the patient activates the pump that pushes insulin through the syringe and tubing and into the body tissue via a subcutaneously inserted needle.

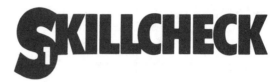

SKILLCHECK

1. Morton O'Reilly, a 40-year-old executive, has been admitted to the CCU because of acute chest pain. After 3 days, he is scheduled for discharge because neither his EKG nor cardiac enzymes show evidence of a myocardial infarction. During hospitalization, though, Mr. O'Reilly has had several fasting blood glucose tests that showed moderate elevation. Should he have a glucose tolerance test before being sent home? Why?

2. Willard Jones is an 85-year-old resident of a nursing home. During a routine physical examination, his blood chemistry profile (fasting) shows his blood glucose to be 130 mg/dl. Do you think he should have a glucose tolerance test?

3. Martha Simon, a 27-year-old salesclerk, takes 4 units of regular insulin and 26 units of NPH insulin every morning. She eats breakfast at 7 a.m. and lunch at noon. On very active days, though, she frequently experiences hypoglycemic reactions around 10 a.m. What would you suggest to alleviate her hypoglycemic episodes?

4. Julie, age 16, takes 8 units of regular insulin and 38 units of NPH. She tries to follow her diet but finds that even when she does, her bedtime Clinitest reads 2%. To compound matters, Julie frequently has hypoglycemic reactions during the night. She has tried to alleviate them by eating a piece of fruit before bed, but this doesn't seem to help. She says she doesn't want to increase her caloric intake by increasing her diet. What could you suggest to Julie?

5. Paul, age 14, is always hungry and eats continuously. He takes 50 units of Lente insulin and has been given a 3,200-calorie diet appropriate to his age, size, and activity. Paul says that all his urine tests read 2% but he can't stop eating and needs huge quantities of food. What alternatives would you investigate?

6. Harold Jefferson, a 52-year-old accountant with a history of hypertension and congestive heart failure, has just been diagnosed as diabetic. He has been taking digoxin (Lanoxin) and hydro-

chlorothiazide (HydroDIURIL) for his other medical conditions: he is allergic to sulfisoxazole (Gantrisin). Would you expect the doctor to place Mr. Jefferson on oral hypoglycemic agents?

7. Jane Scarlotti, a 43-year-old advertising executive, is a Type II diabetic patient who's been on tolbutamide therapy, twice daily, for about 5 years. Although her doctor has been pleased with Ms. Scarlotti's response to the oral hypoglycemic, recent urine tests show that her blood glucose level is not being consistently controlled. Although she claims to take her medication regularly, she admits to "occasionally" forgetting a dose. Her doctor has talked about changing to insulin, but Ms. Scarlotti "hates needles." What other therapy might the doctor consider?

8. Sarah Steinman, a 39-year-old newly diagnosed diabetic patient, has been told to take 42 units of NPH insulin and 7 units of regular insulin. After 2 weeks, she reports wild fluctuations in response to her therapy; some days she has hypoglycemic reactions and other days she feels fine. When she describes her injection technique, it sounds fine. What are some likely causes of the fluctuations?

9. Six months after beginning therapy on oral hypoglycemic agents, Frank Fisher is hospitalized with congestive heart failure. A nursing student notices that Mr. Fisher has diabetes and is being treated with chlorpropamide at home. She asks you why his chlorpropamide hasn't been ordered in the hospital to maintain control. What explanation would you give her?

10. Jacqueline Bond is a "Type A," competitive personality with a responsible job. She takes 44 units of Lente insulin once daily. Although she eats a fairly standard meal for breakfast and dinner, Ms. Bond's lunches vary from nothing at all to a full-course meal with cocktails. She feels that the large lunches are necessary for business. How would you advise Ms. Bond to change her eating habits?

(Answers begin on page 204)

HOW TO INSTRUCT PATIENTS

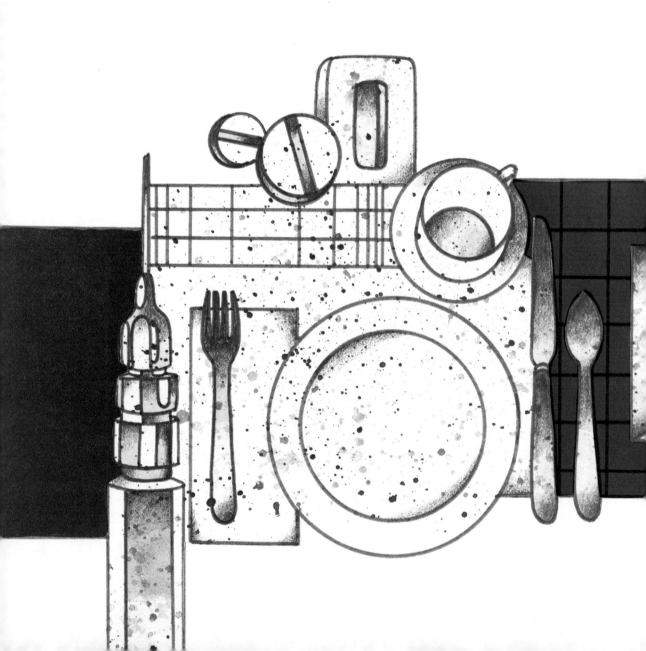

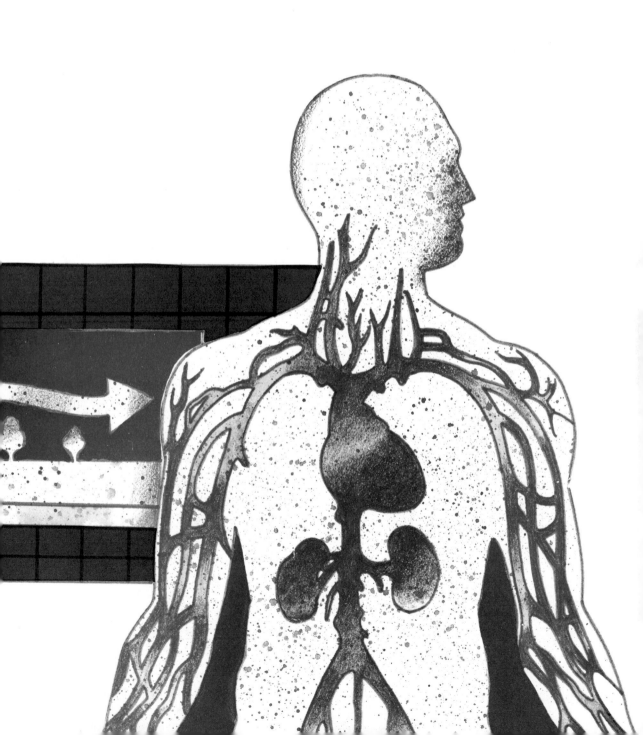

What nursing actions can you take
to prevent ingrown toenails and other
foot problems in a patient with diabetes?

When crossing time zones,
what's the best way to adjust
an insulin management routine?

If your patient is color blind, how can he
obtain an accurate blood glucose reading?

What easy-to-digest foods
help balance insulin and maintain nutrition
during a short-term illness?

6

Helping your patient manage his care

BY VERONICA F. ENGLE, RN

FEW DISEASES DEMAND as much patient participation in therapy as diabetes does. In fact, nearly all persons with diabetes must manage their disease daily by themselves. This places a great deal of responsibility on the person with diabetes, but also places a perhaps more difficult responsibility on you — to work with that person so he can become a knowledgeable, willing manager of his own care.

Many diabetes education programs rely heavily on pre-printed materials that aren't individualized, are difficult to read, and are confusing. This chapter, however, presents *basic* patient education material. In addition to using the materials in this chapter, you should provide handouts that repeat all instructions. Not only will these reinforce what you have taught him, they will also provide him with a handy reference at home. Here are two handout suggestions.

• Develop a very basic pamphlet, suitable for persons with insulin-dependent and non-insulin-dependent diabetes, that compares the human body to a car. As instructor, you would explain that both require fuel (gasoline or food), but to burn the fuel, both need a starter (key or insulin). Use the word ''food'' rather than ''carbohydrate'' to emphasize the importance of the total diet. You could use the car analogy to point out the patient's responsibility in self-care (just as he must care for

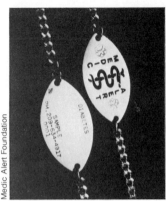

Identify yourself
It is important for persons with
diabetes to carry some kind
of identification, such as these
Medic Alert bracelets, so that
their condition will be treated
properly in an emergency.

Medic Alert Foundation

his car). You also could use the analogy to show that an excess
of glucose (high blood sugar), just like an excess of gasoline,
will spill over and can be measured, and that the body, like a
car, will not run without fuel (low blood sugar).

The next section would contain an illustration of the four
elements that affect the blood glucose level — food, insulin,
exercise, and stress. Use this as a jumping-off point to develop
the patient's conceptual understanding of diabetes management and to develop his problem-solving skills regarding such
questions as: Should he exercise before or after meals? Why
must he eat his meals on time? What will happen if he's sick?

Also included in this section would be a simple chart about
high and low blood glucose levels. It would outline the causes,
quickness of onset, signs (including urine test results), and treatment of both conditions. In discussing this section, emphasize
prevention. To make sure the patient thoroughly understands the
causes and effects of high and low blood glucose levels, refer
back to the problem-solving skills you taught in the last section.
If the patient is taking insulin or oral hypoglycemic agents, explain the differences between the two and make certain he knows
what an insulin reaction is and how to treat it.

Pictures of the right and wrong ways to cut toenails would
come next, reinforcing your visual or photographic program.
Finally, the pamphlet could contain pictures and information
on the types of identification bracelets and necklaces available.
Suggest that the patient select a bracelet, since it is more visible than a necklace. Also suggest that he choose a form of
identification with ''I have diabetes'' printed on it. It is more
apt to catch someone's attention in a crisis than a wallet card.
• The second handout, directed solely at the insulin-
dependent patient, would briefly summarize all the insulin-
related instructions from the educational program: types and
concentrations of insulin, drawing up insulin, giving an injection, urine testing for patients with insulin-dependent diabetes,
adjusting insulin dosages, and self-care during sick days (vital
information that is often neglected). It also could include a
site rotation chart and a chart for recording urine tests. If your
patient is non-insulin-dependent, you should give him a sheet
explaining urine testing and a chart for recording results.
Neither handout need be elaborate. You could make them by
photocopying typed pages and stapling them together.

In addition to the patient-education material, you should

Report of Urine Tests

Patient's full name _____

Type of test(s) _____ Time (s) _____

Date	Urine tests				Medication	Remarks
Month, day, year	Breakfast	Noon	Supper	Bedtime		

have a Diabetes Assessment Sheet for your own use. This sheet would contain all possible topics that you might discuss with the patient and his family. One column should be headed "Assessment," where you could record the results of your initial interview with the patient and the points you'll need to cover with other nursing personnel. Initial and date the second column, "Instruction," when you've covered the education program with the patient. Check the next three columns, "Patient Comprehends," "Patient Demonstrates," and "Family Instructed," when appropriate. Finally, leave a blank space in your assessment sheet where you can record notes. An assessment sheet will keep all of the staff informed about the teaching plan and can be used for a chart audit. Use it while the patient is in the hospital for discharge planning. That way, you'll ensure continuity of care and you can judge how much of his inpatient instructions he has retained.

Throughout your program, remember that teaching aids are not a substitute for your individualized instructions. Rather, you should use them to complement your instructions.

You'll find the information on the following pages helpful. And at the end of the chapter, you'll find a summary of important nursing tips to remember when teaching self-care. Remember that your primary goal is to work with the patient to help him establish his own goals for self-care. Only if he understands and helps establish his daily regimen can you expect knowledgeable and safe self-care from him.

Insulin concentration

Most hospitals use only U-100 insulin, although U-40 is still available for children and U-500 may be used to treat massive insulin resistance.

Insulin concentration refers to the number of units of insulin protein in 1 ml of solution. (U-100 insulin contains 100 units of insulin in 1 ml). Make sure you use only a U-100 syringe with U-100 insulin. The syringe has black and orange markings. The bottle has black letters and an orange cap.

Types of insulin

1 and 1a. There are different types of insulin, such as regular, NPH, or Lente. The insulins act over different periods of time, which may vary from one person to another.

2. The most common rapid-acting insulin is regular insulin. Regular insulin's onset, or when it begins to work, is 20 to 30 minutes after injection; its peak, or when it works best, is 3 to 5 hours; and its duration, or when it is all gone, is 5 to 8 hours.

If you use only regular insulin, you will have to take an injection before each meal.

3. The most common intermediate insulins are NPH and Lente.

NPH insulin's onset is 1 to 1½ hours after injection; its peak is 8 to 12 hours; and its duration is 24 to 28 hours.

Lente insulin's onset is 1 to 1½ hours after injection; its peak is 8 to 12 hours; and its duration is 24 to 28 hours.

With either type of intermediate insulin, you would most likely have an insulin reaction in the late afternoon, when the insulin is peaking. Eat an afternoon snack and carry candy to treat a reaction. Also eat a snack every night to prevent insulin reactions while you sleep.

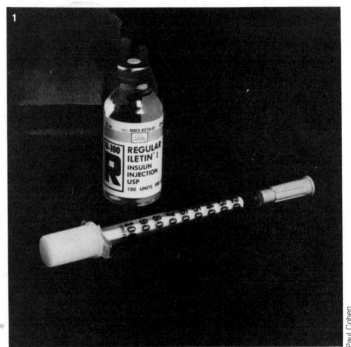

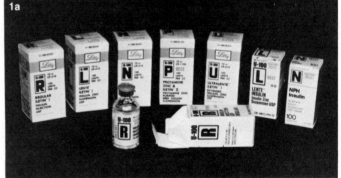

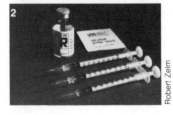

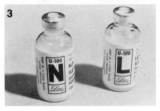

PATIENT-TEACHING AIDS

4. If you use NPH or Lente insulin, you may need only one injection a day. However, some patients need to take two types of insulin: a rapid-acting and an intermediate insulin. For example, you may be taking regular plus NPH insulin. The regular insulin is used because it peaks at noon, and the NPH does not peak until the late afternoon.

Always use the correct type of insulin and know when it acts. Check your insulin before you fill your syringe.

You may store the bottle of insulin you're currently using at room temperature (around 77° F., or 25° C.). Refrigerate extra bottles of insulin, but avoid freezing.

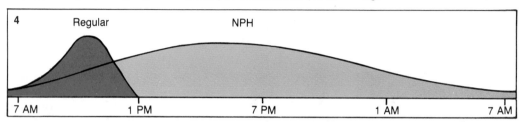

Injection sites

Insulin injections may be given in areas that have a thick layer of fat and are free from large blood vessels and nerves. You may safely use your upper arms, abdomen, thigh, and buttocks.

Do not use the same spot for injection more than once every 2 months. It is important to rotate sites to prevent changes in the fatty tissue that can interfere with the absorption of insulin.

1. Use this chart to help you remember where to give your injection, as well as to record that you gave it.

2. Start with spot A1 for your injection. The next day, use spot A2. Continue using spots A3 to A7 in the same manner.

Next, use the spots on your right abdomen, B1 through B7, as before. In the same manner, use your thighs and buttocks.

You may need to add or subtract spots, depending upon the amount of fat that you have. For example, if you have a large stomach, you can add more spots there.

1	INJECTION SITE							
SITE		1	2	3	4	5	6	7
Right abdomen	A							
Left abdomen	B							
Right thigh	C							
Left thigh	D							
Right arm	E							
Left arm	F							
Right back (below waist)	G							
Left back (below waist)	H							
Right buttock	I							
Left buttock	J							

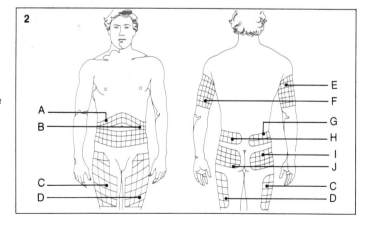

3. Measure the area on your arm with your hand. Place your hand on your shoulder and draw an imaginary line beneath your hand.

4. Place your hand above your elbow and draw an imaginary line above your hand.

5. Use the middle and outer area of your arm between these lines.

6. Measure the area on your thigh with your hand. Place your hand on your knee and draw a line above it. Place your hand on your hip bone and draw a line below it.

7. Use the middle and outer area of your thigh between these lines.

8. Measure the area on your abdomen with your hand. Place your hands on your lower ribs and draw a line.

9. Place your hands on your hip bones and draw a line.

10. Use the area between these two lines, as far around as you can pinch up fat. Do not use the belt line or a 1″ area around your navel.

11. You may also use your buttocks, or upper arms or shoulders if you have enough fat to pinch up.

If you are using an area for the first time, the insulin may be absorbed better and you could have an insulin reaction. Remember to carry candy to treat an insulin reaction.

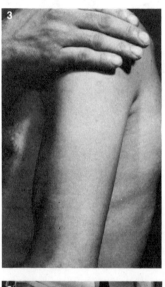

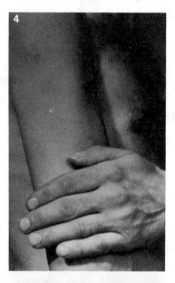

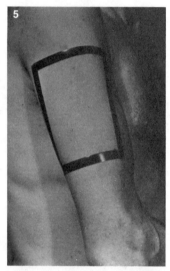

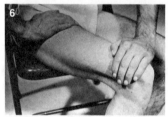

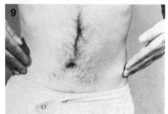

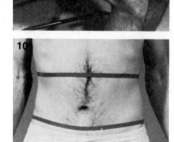

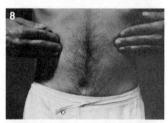

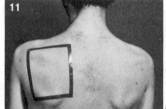

Photos by Robert Zelm

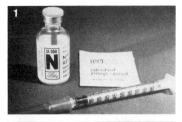

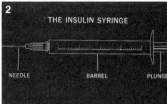

THE INSULIN SYRINGE

NEEDLE   BARREL   PLUNGE

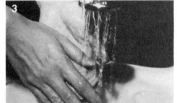

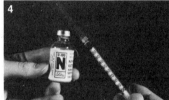

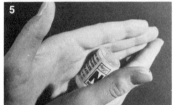

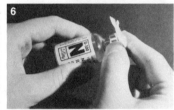

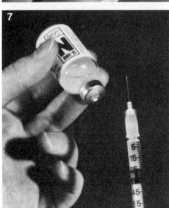

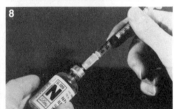

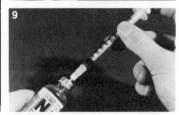

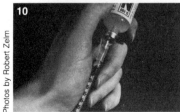

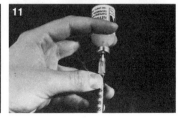

Photos by Robert Zelm

Drawing up insulin

1. This is the equipment that you will need to draw up insulin, or put insulin into the syringe. You will need a sterile syringe and needle, insulin, and an alcohol swab.

2. You cannot touch the needle because it will enter the body. You *can* touch the barrel and the plunger of the syringe.

3. Wash your hands. This is *always* the first step.

4. Assemble your equipment in a clean area. Check that the insulin and syringe match. If you are using U-100 insulin, you must use a U-100 syringe. Also check that you have the correct type of insulin.

5. Roll the bottle of insulin between your hands to mix it. Mix gently to prevent large air bubbles in the insulin. A white layer may form at the bottom of the bottle of insulin; this must be mixed.

6. Scrub the top of the bottle with an alcohol swab. You may also use a cotton ball and rubbing alcohol.

7. Pull the plunger out to the same number of units of insulin that you will take out. This will pull air into the syringe. Take off the needle cover. The needle cover protects the needle from touching anything.

8. Put the needle into the rubber on top of the bottle of insulin.

9. Push the plunger in. This will push air into the bottle and prevent a vacuum.

10. Hold the bottle and syringe together. Turn them upside down. The bottle is now on top. You may hold the bottle between your thumb and forefinger, while holding the syringe between your ring and little fingers, against the palm of your hand.

11. You may also hold the bottle between your forefinger and middle finger, while holding the syringe between your thumb and little finger.

12. Pull back on the plunger to the correct number of units of insulin.

13. Check for air bubbles. (Air is clear. NPH and Lente insulin are cloudy; regular insulin is clear.) Air bubbles will not harm you, *but* they may prevent you from taking the correct amount of insulin.

14. Remove air bubbles by pulling the plunger further out. Push the plunger back to the correct number of units of insulin. This will push the air back into the bottle. (You may not be able to remove all of the tiny air bubbles.)

15. You also may flick the barrel of the syringe sharply with your middle finger.

16. Or, you may push the plunger back in. This will push the air and insulin back into the bottle. Pull the plunger out again to the correct number of units of insulin.

Check that the syringe contains the correct amount of insulin and there are no air bubbles. If there are no bubbles and the correct amount of insulin is in the syringe, take the needle out of the bottle.

17. Put the cover back on the needle. This will protect the needle until you are ready to give yourself the injection.

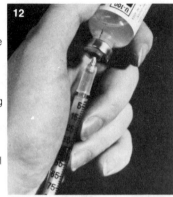

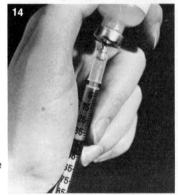

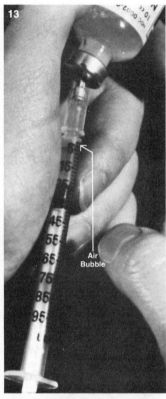

Air Bubble

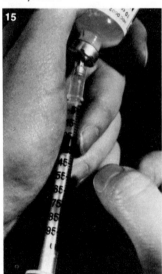

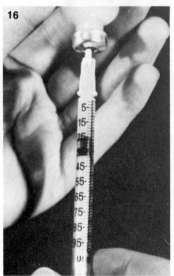

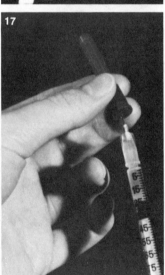

Photos by Robert Zelm

PATIENT-TEACHING AIDS

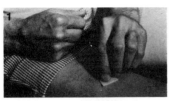

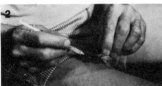

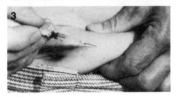

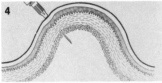

Injecting insulin
Use your injection chart to find the spot where you will give yourself the injection of insulin.

1. Wipe off the spot with an alcohol swab or use alcohol on a cotton ball.

2. Take the cover off the needle and put it aside temporarily. Hold the syringe like a pencil.

3. Grasp the spot where you will give the injection between the thumb and fingers of your free hand. Pinch up firmly!

To pinch up the spot on your arm, press the back of your upper arm against a chair back or corner of a wall. "Roll" your arm down.

4. Pinching up the spot will pull the fat away from the muscle. The injection will be into the fat.

5. Put the needle into the spot with a jab, like throwing a dart. Do not *push* the needle in. If your syringe has a long needle, insert it at a 45° angle, all the way to the end of the needle.

6. You may also spread the skin between your fingers and insert the needle straight up and down. Use this technique if you have more fat. If you're using a syringe with a short (½") needle, insert it straight into the skin.

7. *Optional step:* Let go of the spot and use that hand to pull back on the plunger about two units. Check for blood near the needle. If there isn't any, push the plunger in. If you see blood, the needle is in a small blood vessel. Pull the needle out and put it into another spot, as before. Check again; if there is no blood, push the plunger in. If you see blood, pull the needle out and throw away the syringe. Draw up a new syringe of insulin and use this for your injection.

8. Push in the plunger.

9. Place the alcohol swab over the needle after you have pushed the plunger in. Pull the needle out quickly and press the swab over the spot for 2 seconds: do not rub. Put the cover on the needle.

10. Break the needle off by quickly snapping the syringe and needle together, like breaking a stick. Throw away the syringe and needle. Write on the chart where you took the injection.

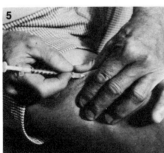

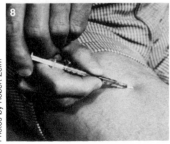

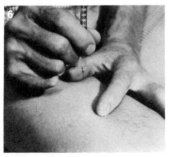

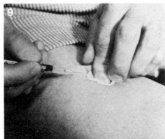

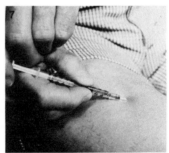

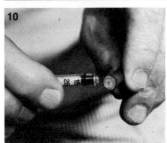

Daily foot care

As you grow older, the circulation to your feet decreases. This is especially true for the diabetic patient. With decreased circulation, your body can't heal injuries to your feet. An ingrown toenail or blister can lead to an infection. The nerves in your feet that tell you if something is too hot or too cold may also be affected. You may burn yourself and not know it. So, taking care of your feet every day is important to prevent foot problems.

Always take care of your feet at the same time every day. Choose the time of day that is best for you.

1. You will need the following equipment: a basin, washcloth and towel, mild soap, shoes, and socks. You may also use a bathtub or shower.

2. Wash your feet in water that's 90° to 95° F. (32° to 35° C.). To prevent burns, always check the temperature of the water with your hand or elbow before putting your feet in.

3. Soak your feet for 5 to 10 minutes.

4. Use a soapy washcloth to wash your whole foot, especially between your toes and around your toenails.

5. Dry your feet gently but thoroughly with a towel, especially between your toes.

6. If you have dry skin, it may look like this.

7. Apply a lotion to your feet immediately after washing and before drying. This will prevent the water from evaporating and drying your skin. The lotion will keep your skin soft.

If you have sweaty feet, use a mild foot powder or cornstarch. Put it between your toes, in your socks, and in your shoes.

8. Inspect your feet every day for injuries. This is just as important as washing your feet. With decreased feeling in your feet, you may not feel an injury. Inju-

ries include pressure from shoes that are too tight, a cut on a toe, or stepping on a tack. Look between your toes, around the toenails, and at every part of your foot for cracks, blisters, corns, calluses, and red and swollen areas. If you find an injury, wash the area with warm, soapy water. You may use a mild antiseptic, such as Bactine, but don't use harsh antiseptics, such as iodine. Do not use your injured foot. Elevate it as often as possible. This will help the circulation to heal the injury.

If an injury becomes infected, it will be red, swollen, painful, and hot, and may ooze pus. Call your doctor *immediately* if an injury doesn't heal or becomes infected.

9. You can also injure yourself by cutting corns and calluses or using a liquid corn remover. You may cut too deeply or the corn remover may burn too deeply. If you have corns and calluses, rub them with a towel after washing your feet. If necessary, consult a podiatrist.

10. Wear clean socks every

day. Cotton or wool socks absorb perspiration best. Socks should be smooth and have loose tops. A tight top could cut off circulation to your feet. You may wear either white socks or colored socks, as long as the dye is colorfast.

Always wear leather shoes. (Leather shoes allow your feet to "breathe"; plastic shoes cause your feet to perspire and can lead to fungal infections, blisters, and rashes.) Make sure your shoes have ties or buckles with a low heel and are properly fitted. Buy them at the end of the day, when your feet will be the largest. Break in new shoes gradually, wearing them ½ hour a day. If possible, have several pairs and wear a different pair each day.

Before putting on your shoes, check inside them for objects, rough spots, or torn linings, which could injure your feet.

Never go barefoot or wear shoes without socks. Socks and shoes protect your feet from injury.

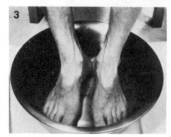

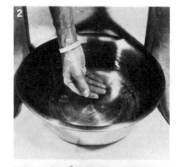

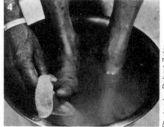

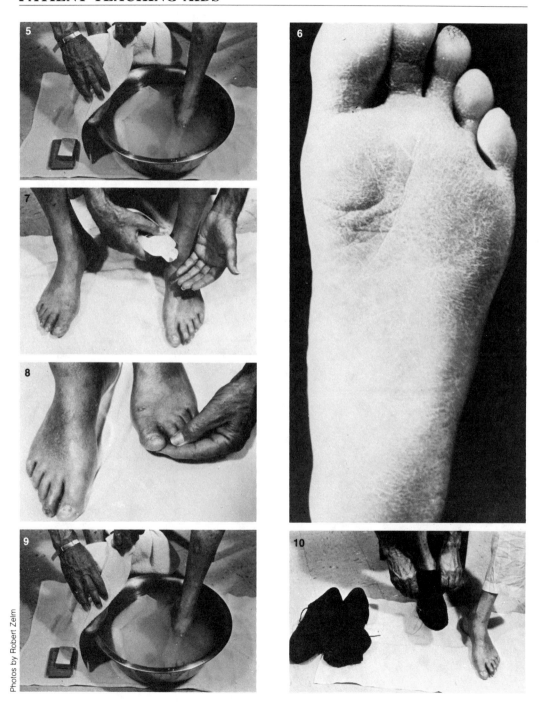

Cutting toenails

Many people have difficulty cutting their toenails. Their toenails may be thick, tough, or misshapen. Or they may have difficulty seeing or reaching their toenails to cut them safely. If you have any of these difficulties, ask a member of your family, a nurse, or a doctor to cut your toenails for you, or see a podiatrist.

1. This is the equipment that you will need: a basin, towel, emery board, and nippers, scissors, or a clipper with a straight edge.

2. Soak your feet in warm water. Check the temperature of the water with your hand or elbow before putting your feet in. Soak your feet for 15 to 20 minutes. This will soften your toenails. Dry your feet gently, but thoroughly, by blotting them with a towel. (You may want to cut your toenails during your daily foot care, after washing and drying your feet.)

3. When cutting, use only the end of the nipper or scissors blade. This will prevent splitting of the nail.

4. Take short "bites" across the nail. Start at the corner, cutting the nail straight across, even with the end of the toe.

5. If you cut into the corners, you may cut a hook that will dig into the toe as the nail grows. Likewise, if you cut the nail too short, it will also dig into the toe as the nail grows.

6. File any ragged edge with an emery board. This will prevent the toenails from digging into adjacent toes and from tearing the stockings. If you can't cut your toenails because they are thick and tough, file your toenails with an emery board every day after washing and drying your feet. This will prevent the need to cut your toenails.

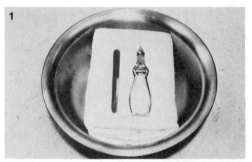

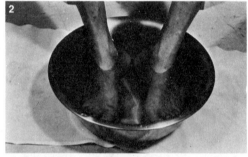

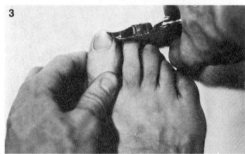

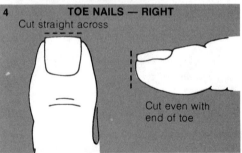

TOE NAILS — RIGHT
Cut straight across
Cut even with end of toe

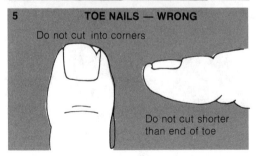

TOE NAILS — WRONG
Do not cut into corners
Do not cut shorter than end of toe

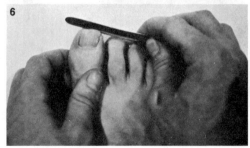

Photos by Robert Zelm

PATIENT-TEACHING AIDS

Urine testing
Such products as Tes-Tape, Clinistix, and Diastix test the urine for glucose; Keto-Diastix tests the urine for ketones as well as for glucose. You may find ketones in urine if you are losing weight, if you are sick, or if you have very high blood glucose levels.

1. The color chart for a urine test is on the product container. For a Diastix or Keto-Diastix glucose test, the blue color indicates no glucose (negative) and the dark brown color indicates a large amount of glucose (2%). Clinistix and Tes-Tape have similar color charts that indicate the percentage of glu-cose in the urine measuring a range of 0% to 2% glucose. For a Keto-Diastix ketone test, the buff color indicates no ketones (negative) and the dark purple color indicates a large amount of ketones. *Note:* Because color charts differ between products, check to be sure you're using the correct chart.

2. All urine test strips are affected by humidity and sunlight. Always keep the bottle tightly capped, and store it out of direct sunlight. Be sure to check the expiration date on the bottle to guarantee that the strips are fresh.

3. Remove a strip from the bottle; tightly close the cap.

4. To test urine, hold the strip at the end that doesn't have the color blocks, making sure that the printing is facing you. Do not touch the color blocks.

5. Dip the strip into the container of urine for at least 2 seconds. The color blocks must be thoroughly wet. Take the strip out of the urine. Tap the strip against the side of the container to remove excess urine. Begin timing.

6. When using Keto-Diastix, compare the buff color with the ketone color chart *exactly 15 seconds* after removing the strip from the urine. Read the color blocks *only* from the side with the printing. (The glue on the back of the blocks interferes with the test.)

7. When using Diastix or Keto-Diastix, compare the blue color block with the glucose color chart *exactly 30 seconds* after removing the strip from the urine. The color may change after 30 seconds, but ignore it. Remember, record the color *only* at 30 seconds.

8. Record your urine test results every day and bring them with you when you see your nurse or doctor.

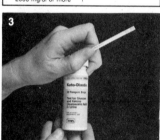

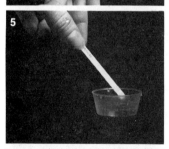

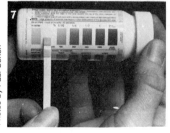

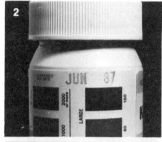

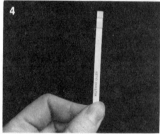

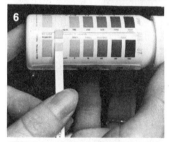

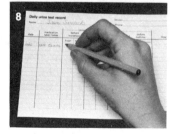

Photos by Paul Cohen

Testing "double-voided" urine
Whenever you test your urine, be sure to test a "double-voided" specimen — that is, urine that has just been filtered by the kidneys. To obtain a double-voided urine specimen, follow these steps:
• Urinate (this will rid your body of all urine).
• Drink a glass of water.
• Urinate again 30 minutes later into a clean container.
• Test the second urine specimen.

Urine testing tips for insulin-dependent diabetes

If you are controlling your diabetes by diet and insulin, test your urine for *glucose* four times a day. Test it before breakfast, lunch, dinner, and bedtime. (As each urine test product has different characteristics, discuss the advantages and disadvantages of each product with your nurse or doctor.)

Always write down your urine test results. Use a record of them to adjust your insulin, diet, and exercise. Bring this record with you when you see your doctor or nurse.

Test your urine four times a day for glucose and ketones when:
• your urine is 1% or 2%.
• you are having signs of high blood glucose, such as excessive thirst, urination, or fatigue.
• you are under physical stress, such as a cold or the flu.
Call your doctor when:
• your urine stays at 1% or 2% for 2 days.
• your urine contains even a small amount of ketones.

Urine testing tips for non-insulin-dependent diabetes

If you are controlling your diabetes by diet, or by diet and medication, test your urine for *glucose* once a day, about 2 hours after the largest meal of the day. Write down your urine test results. Bring a record of them when you see your doctor or nurse.

Your urine should always test negative.

Test your urine four times a day for glucose when:
• your urine is 1% or 2%.
• you are having signs of high blood glucose, such as excessive thirst, urination, or fatigue.
• you are under physical stress, such as a cold or the flu.
Call your doctor if:
• your urine tests are 1% or 2% for 2 days.

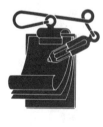

Remember these important points about patient participation in diabetes therapy:
1. Use an assessment sheet to track your patient's progress.
2. Work with your patient to develop a urine-testing schedule that will help him monitor his diabetes.
3. Teach your patient about insulin types, appropriate injection sites, and the prevention and treatment of insulin reactions.
4. Emphasize the importance of proper foot care.

7

Refining
home test tactics

BY DELORES SCHUMANN, RN, MS, FAAN

UNTIL THE RECENT introduction of a method for patient testing of blood glucose levels at home, testing urine for glycosuria was universally used. Now, however, the new method — known as capillary blood glucose monitoring — is recommended for insulin-dependent diabetic patients. This is because it provides accurate information on blood glucose levels when checked at different times during the day.

But this doesn't mean that *every* diabetic patient should make the switch to capillary blood glucose monitoring. In fact, a diabetic patient whose metabolic control of his illness is satisfactory (blood glucose level less than 180 mg/dl) needn't have his routine disrupted. And testing urine is the method of choice for the non-insulin-dependent diabetic patient; this patient needs only an index to his degree of metabolic control — not exact readings of his blood glucose levels.

Test for glycosuria

Like many nurses, you may find urine tests for glycosuria a snap to perform. Yet studies suggest that many nurses neglect to pass along the fine points of urine testing to their patients.

The preceding chapter graphically showed how a patient should conduct a urine test. But to help ensure that he gets accurate test results, you also should explain these ''refine-

Scheduling glycosuria testing
The information below is a handy
reference for determining the
best time to test for glycosuria
and to accurately assess insulin
effectiveness.

Insulin type: Intermediate, taken
   before breakfast
Best urine testing time:
   Before supper

Insulin type: Short-acting, taken
   before breakfast
Best urine testing time:
   Before lunch

Insulin type: Intermediate, taken
   before supper
Best urine testing time:
   Before breakfast

Insulin type: Short-acting, taken
   before supper
Best urine testing time:
   Before going to bed

ments'' of urine testing.

Glycosuria, the presence of glucose in the urine, depends on two things: the plasma glucose level and the renal threshold (the point of blood glucose concentration at which the kidney excretes glucose). Normally, glycosuria doesn't occur until plasma glucose concentration exceeds the renal threshold. In most patients, this occurs at a plasma glucose level of 160 to 180 mg/dl. But you should be aware of the exceptions. Diabetic patients (particularly the younger and the well-controlled) and elderly persons, who have elevated renal thresholds, could have negative urine tests even though their plasma glucose is high. Conversely, an occasional diabetic patient will have a low renal threshold. He'll test positive to glycosuria even though his plasma glucose isn't elevated.

Glycosuria tests consist of two main types: reducing and enzyme. Reducing tests (for example, Clinitest, Benedict's test) react with sugars other than glucose. That is, they develop a positive reaction if galactose, lactose, maltose, or pentose is present in the urine. Enzyme tests (for example, Tes-Tape, Clinistix, Diastix) respond specifically to glucose by producing a color change on a paper strip or stick.

You should be aware of the basic differences between these tests to choose the appropriate one for your diabetic patient. For example, nursing mothers and women in their third trimester of pregnancy have lactose in their urine, so they should use an enzyme test, such as Tes-Tape, because it checks only for glucose.

With the enzyme tests, the patient compares the color change on the test strip with a reference color chart supplied by the manufacturer. Be sure to assess your patient's color vision before proceeding. (Make sure he uses only charts with bright colors; faded color charts won't allow him to distinguish adequately between color sequences.)

The color charts distributed by the various manufacturers aren't interchangeable. For example, the color sequences on the charts for Clinitest and Tes-Tape are just the reverse of each other — orange indicates a negative response to Tes-Tape, but it suggests a 2% concentration of glucose for Clinitest.

Until recently, all glucose oxidase tests used the plus (+) symbol to indicate glycosuria. But lack of standardization of what the use of the symbol meant, from product to product,

Substances Affecting Urine Test Results

URINE CONSTITUENTS
high specific gravity
- *Clinistix*

Depresses color development
- *Diastix*

No effect
- *Tes-Tape*

No effect
- *Clinitest*

No effect

low specific gravity
- *Clinistix*

Intensifies color development
- *Diastix*

No effect
- *Tes-Tape*

No effect
- *Clinitest*

No effect

creatinine
- *Clinistix*

No effect
- *Diastix*

No effect
- *Tes-Tape*

No effect
- *Clinitest*

No effect

uric acid
- *Clinistix*

No effect
- *Diastix*

No effect
- *Tes-Tape*

No effect
- *Clinitest*

No effect

ketone bodies
- *Clinistix*

No effect
- *Diastix*

May affect color development when ingested in large amounts
- *Tes-Tape*

No effect
- *Clinitest*

No effect

DRUGS
ascorbic acid (vitamin C)
- *Clinistix*

May cause false-negative reading
- *Diastix*

May cause low reading when ingested in large amounts
- *Tes-Tape*

May interfere with color formation when ingested in large amounts
- *Clinitest*

May cause false reading when ingested in large amounts

Levodopa
- *Clinistix*

Large concentration may cause false-negative reading
- *Diastix*

Large concentration may cause false-negative reading
- *Tes-Tape*

No effect
- *Clinitest*

No effect

cephalosporins
- *Clinistix*

No effect
- *Diastix*

No effect
- *Tes-Tape*

No effect
- *Clinitest*

May cause false-positive reading

nalidixic acid
- *Clinistix*

No effect
- *Diastix*

No effect
- *Tes-Tape*

No effect
- *Clinitest*

May cause false-positive reading

probenecid
- *Clinistix*

No effect
- *Diastix*

No effect
- *Tes-Tape*

No effect
- *Clinitest*

May cause false-positive reading

Pyridium
- *Clinistix*

No effect
- *Diastix*

Masks color reactions
- *Tes-Tape*

No effect
- *Clinitest*

No effect

salicylates
- *Clinistix*

No effect
- *Diastix*

May give low reading when ingested in large amounts
- *Tes-Tape*

No effect
- *Clinitest*

May give false-positive reading when ingested in large amounts

SUBSTANCES AFFECTING KETONE TESTS
Levodopa
- *Ketostix*

Causes false-positive reading
- *Acetest*

Causes false-positive reading

bromsulphalein (BSP)
- *Ketostix*

Causes false-positive reading
- *Acetest*

Causes false-positive reading

salicylate, or aspirin metabolites
- *Ketostix*

No effect
- *Acetest*

No effect

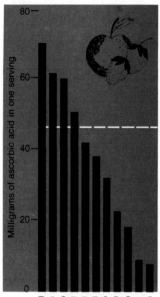

Watch out for Vitamin C!
In the above chart, the dotted line represents the recommended daily allowance of ascorbic acid. A high amount of vitamin C in the diet can give false-negative urine test results. With Clinistix, if there is 0.1% glucose in the patient's urine, between 10 to 20 mg/dl of vitamin C can give a false-negative reading. Warn your patient to keep an eye on how much vitamin C he ingests. If your patient questions the accuracy of his urine test and has been consuming large quantities of vitamin C, suggest that he retest with Diastix or Clinitest, which is less sensitive to vitamin C.

made regulation of insulin dosages difficult. As a result, some manufacturers have stopped using the plus symbol and use the glucose percentage instead. Note: Results for Clinistix, however, are reported as negative, light, medium, or dark.

To ensure accuracy in the hospital, you should record urine test results by the percentage of glucose present rather than by pluses. And most important — be sure to specify which test was used. If you test a patient with Clinitest tablets and the evening nurse uses Tes-Tape, determining the exact amount of glucose the patient is excreting becomes impossible. And the inconsistency in test results would cause erratic regulation of insulin dosage.

How drugs affect glycosuria tests
Drugs containing sugar. If a diabetic patient begins to show glucose in his urine after he has started taking a new medication, he should check to see whether that drug contains sugar and, if so, the type of sugar. Many medicinal agents contain sweeteners, flavoring agents, or fillers that have a high sugar content. Elixirs, suspensions, and syrups (for example, cough syrups, antibiotic suspensions) often have sugar as part of their base. If a diabetic patient takes these drugs, he may ingest a substantially higher amount of carbohydrate than his prescribed diet allows. The added glucose intake will, of course, show up in his glycosuria test.

Ascorbic acid and aspirin. Diabetic patients who consume large quantities of ascorbic acid (vitamin C) or aspirin should know that these drugs produce metabolites that cause misleading test results. Since ascorbic acid and aspirin are used so widely and with relative safety, they're not often thought of as problem sources.

Large quantities of vitamin C can creep into a diet in subtle ways. Because this vitamin is popularly credited with such a wide range of therapeutic properties, even a diabetic patient who's aware of the restrictions imposed on his diet might take it. For instance, he might take multiple vitamin or iron preparations, which contain varying amounts of vitamin C, without his doctor's recommendation or knowledge. Or he could be getting large amounts of this vitamin from fruits, fruit drinks, or foods that have been fortified with vitamin C as the food preservative and antioxidant. Still another source is intravenous tetracycline preparations, which are buffered with ascorbic acid.

Aspirin produces false-positive glycosuria test results through the metabolite gentisic acid. Since only about 1% to 8% of aspirin is converted to gentisic acid, a casual dose wouldn't affect test results. But 2.4 g, or seven tablets, of aspirin per day *could* produce enough gentisic acid in the urine to affect the measurement of glycosuria. This means that patients who take aspirin regularly — for arthritis, for instance — can have enough gentisic acid to affect urine tests.

Other affecting drugs. A diabetic patient should always be sure to check the manufacturer's insert packaged with the test materials to see which specific drugs are known to affect test results. Clinitest, for example, will indicate false-positive results if he is taking sufficient concentrations of nalidixic acid (NegGram), cephalosporin antibiotics (Keflin, Keflex), probenecid (Benemid), or vitamin C (ascorbic acid). Drugs known to alter results with Tes-Tape are levodopa (Dopar, Larodopa), methyldopa (Aldomet), aspirin, and ascorbic acid. If a patient is taking any of these medications, he should ask his doctor to switch him to a urine test that isn't affected by the medication.

Urine specimens

Although in the past a Type I (insulin-dependent) diabetic patient always used a second-voided urine specimen for glycosuria testing, research now shows that a first-voided specimen may produce more accurate results. In fact, researchers say that the amount of glucose in a first-voided specimen is equal to or greater than the amount found in the second-voided specimen. One reason for this may be the fact that the patient may need to drink a large quantity of fluid in order to void a second time.

However, a second-voided urine specimen may be requested when the doctor wants to establish a patient's renal threshold for glucose or when:
• a simultaneous plasma glucose level is needed
• a before-breakfast level is needed for a patient taking intermediate or long-acting insulin
• a patient is taking additional insulin because of illness.

The results of a second-voided specimen reflect the patient's current blood glucose levels and should be used to determine if he needs additional regular insulin. To obtain a second-voided urine specimen, have the patient empty his bladder of

Reliability tests
A patient can detect deterioration in some test materials by a change in the color of the agent (for example, Tes-Tape becomes brown, while Clinitest tablets change from a robin's egg blue to a dark, speckled color and eventually to black). But a test agent can deteriorate without changing color. So if he has any reason to suspect its reliability, he should check it in a glucose solution. The test material should give a reading of 2% or more glucose. A "suitable glucose solution" might be a freshly opened bottle or can of cola that contains sugar. Make sure the patient knows not to use dietetic colas, though, as their glucose content differs from that of regular colas. Table sugar is not suitable for this purpose, either, since it is sucrose, not glucose.

Monitoring blood glucose at home

Blood glucose monitoring at home now allows many patients to determine blood glucose levels daily as they work toward maintaining their blood glucose at normal or near-normal levels. The Dextro system, a commonly available method of monitoring blood glucose, uses Dextrostix reagent strips and a battery-powered meter known as a reflectance photometer. To monitor blood glucose using this method, follow these steps:

1. Have your patient perform a fingerstick, and place the second drop of blood on the reagent strip, as shown.

2. Instruct him to wait 1 minute, then wash the blood off the strip with a steady stream of water.

3. If he's not using a reflectance photometer, at this point have him compare the test-block color with the bottle's color chart. Normal results range from 45 to 130 mg/dl. Show him how to document the results.

4. If the patient is using a reflectance photometer, show him how to position the strip — test block side down — in the meter. Then, have him press the READ button.

Within a few seconds, expect to see the glucose level reading appear on the display screen. Emphasize to your patient the importance of documenting the results.

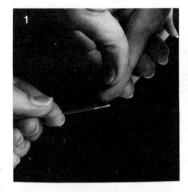

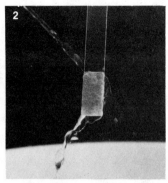

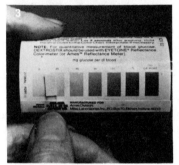

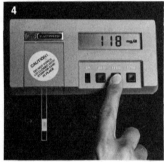

all urine, drink some water, and void again about a half hour later — providing the glycosuria test specimen.

Misuse of test materials

A diabetic patient should never use test materials that have a past expiration date, are discolored, or have been exposed to moisture. Moisture, perhaps more than anything else, causes deterioration of test materials.

The patient's handling of test materials is important. He shouldn't leave Tes-Tape strips lying on utility room sinks, bathroom shelves, or near water faucets. Nor should he leave tablet and enzyme-strip bottles uncovered from one test time to the next. Since most test materials come in jars with screw-top lids and a desiccant to minimize moisturizing effects, he must be sure to use them. He can protect the Tes-Tape dispenser by keeping it in a small jar with a screw-top lid between uses.

The patient must always read the directions accompanying the test materials and follow them precisely. For example, he must hold a Tes-Tape strip in the air during the reaction. If he lays it on a piece of paper, small amounts of glucose from the paper could affect the results. And he should *never* dip the strip in urine and then blot the excess by brushing it against a paper towel.

Be sure he knows that he must wait the specified length of time before he reads the test results. This is especially important with Clinitest, which may use a one-, two-, or five-drop method. With the one- and two-drop methods, glucose levels can be quantitated as high as 10%, whereas the five-drop method only measures to 2%. The patient must watch the Clinitest reaction during its entire process, though, and for 15 seconds after it stops boiling inside the tube, to obtain accurate results. If the color of the specimen in the five-drop method changes rapidly from green to tan to orange to a dark greenish brown (this is known as pass-through color change), the urine has a glucose concentration greater than 2%. The patient shouldn't try to compare these results with the regular color chart. If he is using the two-drop method, be sure that he has the special color chart for it. Make sure, too, that he:

• handles the reagent tablet without touching it — to avoid contaminating it or burning his hand or fingers

• stores the tablets in a place inaccessible to children, who might ingest them and suffer esophageal burns and strictures

• stores the tablets away from other medications, so no one will mistake the test tablets for another drug (such as aspirin) and suffer injury by ingesting some of them.

Testing for ketone bodies

There are three types of ketone bodies — beta hydroxybutyric acid (the most prevalent), acetoacetate, and acetone — and small amounts of these may normally be present in the urine. Like glucose, however, ketones are usually excreted into the urine only after they reach a threshold level in the blood.

Ketonuria occurs not only in diabetic patients but also in nondiabetic persons as a result of reducing diets or eating a high-fat, high-protein, low-carbohydrate diet. Fasting, pregnancy, lactation, and severe infections accompanied by vomiting and diarrhea can cause positive results in ketone tests. On the other hand, severe dehydration or advanced kidney disease may produce a high level of ketone bodies in the blood, but the amount excreted into the urine won't reflect the excessive level.

To test for ketone bodies, a freshly voided urine specimen is required. This is because urine that stands at room temper-

Tips for interpreting glucose oxidase tests
When you teach your patient how to record and interpret the results of his glucose oxidase tests, be sure to stress these two points:
• When he records his test results, tell him to take care to note any special information that may alter them — for example, an insulin reaction, a change in eating patterns, altered activity or exercise patterns, or presence of an infection. This information helps to explain occasional glycosuria and to detect hypoglycemia; it also may suggest modification in the diet plan and insulin therapy.
• Remind your patient that the pattern of results from a series of tests is more valuable than the results of a single test. Caution him to not become overly concerned about a single test result.

Selecting the right test
When you select a testing method for your patient's self-use, remember that no test will fit all situations. First, assess the patient's health history as well as his ability to manage his condition. Then select a method that he can perform correctly. Finally, check the medications that can affect this test and find out whether your patient is taking any of them. If so, you'll need to either select a different test or warn the patient not to continue taking the medications.

ature stimulates bacterial growth, causing changes in the amount of ketones.

Although ketonuria is a warning signal for the diabetic patient that control of his condition is wavering, it doesn't necessarily indicate impending ketoacidosis. For safety's sake, then, when should the diabetic check for ketones? If he shows negative or trace amounts of glucose in his urine, he needn't check routinely for ketone bodies. But he should check for ketones if he begins to show a concentration of 3/4% or more — or according to many specialists, a 2% (4 +) concentration more than two times in succession or during illness. He should continue this testing every 3 to 4 hours until the ketone bodies are no longer present.

Routine testing for ketone bodies should be done by diabetic patients who (1) haven't attained good control; (2) experience weight loss or stress due to vigorous exercise, exposure to cold, digestive disturbances, surgery, or illness; or (3) are newly diagnosed and whose health status needs to be assessed. Also, you should encourage the patient with insulin-dependent diabetes to check for ketones occasionally, so he doesn't forget the techniques of the testing method.

Remind the patient to observe the same test material precautions that apply to glycosuria tests (see page 80).

Remember these important points about home test tactics:
1. Be aware that a high ascorbic acid (vitamin C) intake can produce misleading urine test results.
2. Familiarize your patient with common misuses of test materials: leaving Tes-Tape strips near water, leaving tablet bottles and enzyme-strip bottles uncovered, laying Tes-Tape on paper or blotting it on a paper towel, and not waiting the specified time before reading the results.
3. Recommend testing for ketone bodies for those patients who haven't attained good control; those who've experienced weight loss or stress due to vigorous exercise, exposure to cold, digestive disturbances, surgery, or illness; or those who've been newly diagnosed and are awaiting assessment of their health status.
4. Consider blood glucose self-monitoring a reliable method of recording daily glucose fluctuations.
5. When selecting a test method for your patient, assess his health history and his ability to manage his condition. Also check if any medication he's taking will affect test results.

8

Explaining axioms for sick days

BY JUDITH C. PETROKAS, RN

MILD, SEEMINGLY UNIMPORTANT illnesses, such as diarrhea or gastrointestinal upset, pose no serious threat to normally healthy people. But such illnesses can pose serious problems to diabetic patients — particularly those patients with insulin-dependent diabetes — because they affect food intake, which affects insulin needs.

Consider, for example, what happened to Mrs. Armstrong, a newly diagnosed diabetic patient who came down with the flu. Since she couldn't tolerate any food and feared having an insulin reaction, she decided to omit her insulin. Feeling too ill to test her urine, she failed to notice her elevated blood glucose level and the appearance of ketones in her urine.

After 8 hours without food or insulin, Mrs. Armstrong became short of breath, very tired, and excessively thirsty and experienced more nausea, vomiting, and frequent urination. In fact, she felt so ill that she asked her neighbor, Mrs. Ryan, to take her to the hospital. The outcome: She was admitted with diabetic ketoacidosis.

All this could have been prevented if Mrs. Armstrong had followed a few simple guidelines on how to take care of herself during a sudden, short-term illness. But her experience wasn't unique — many insulin-dependent diabetic patients make the mistake of not eating and not taking insulin when they become

Sick-day diet
On the opposite page you will find some of the recommended foods your patient can eat when sick to maintain adequate nutrition and balance his insulin. Ginger ale, fruit juices, skim milk, cream soups, egg nog, popsicles, sherbet, ice cream, and Jello are easily digested and gentle on the stomach.

ill. And they end up being hospitalized. An important aspect of working with all diabetic patients, therefore, is to teach them how to cope with short-term illness without sacrificing control of their diabetes.

Defining a short-term illness

The first step is to help patients distinguish between short-term and long-term illnesses. For the diabetic patient, a short-term illness is one in which the acute phase doesn't persist longer than 48 hours (for example, influenza, cold, diarrhea). Or, if it does persist, the patient can tolerate most of the meat exchanges of his prescribed diet, plus all of the fruit, vegetable, and bread exchanges. A long-term illness is one that persists longer than 48 hours (for example, complications arise or the patient shows no improvement after this time). A diabetic patient who has a long-term illness should see his doctor.

Following are some simple guidelines for short-term illnesses. Be sure to explain the importance of each one and tell your patient how he can apply common sense to it.

• *Never omit insulin.* The insulin-dependent diabetic patient (like Mrs. Armstrong) may fear an insulin reaction because he's unable to take his usual amount of food. So, he may decide not to take his insulin or any food except small amounts of fluids. Therefore, you must impress upon him the fact that his body *needs* insulin, despite his decreased food intake.

Explain that his doctor may instruct him to use a sliding scale for regular or rapid-acting insulin when he is ill. But he must not make *any other changes* in his insulin without first consulting his doctor. (If your patient is taking oral agents, he shouldn't try to adjust his dosage during an illness. Tell him to simply stop taking the medication if he can't eat; otherwise, he should take them as usual.)

Also, tell the patient if he vomits or has diarrhea, he should notify his doctor at once. Since vomiting and diarrhea deplete body fluids, causing electrolyte imbalance, these conditions must be corrected as soon as possible.

• *Go to bed and keep warm.* Tell the patient to have someone stay with him if at all possible. If he should have an insulin reaction, having someone there who knows what to do can probably prevent it from becoming severe.

• *Monitor urine glucose levels at least four times a day, using Clinitest reagent tablets.* This rule applies not only to insulin-

10 GM OF CARBOHYDRATE

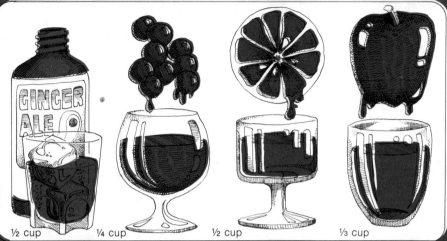

½ cup   ¼ cup   ½ cup   ⅓ cup

12 GM OF CARBOHYDRATE

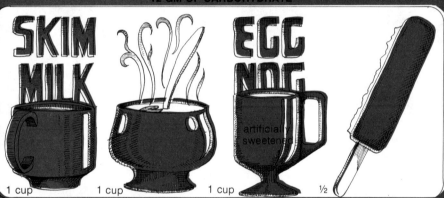

1 cup   1 cup   1 cup   ½

15 GM OF CARBOHYDRATE

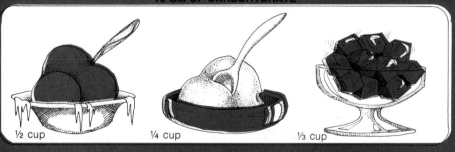

½ cup   ¼ cup   ⅓ cup

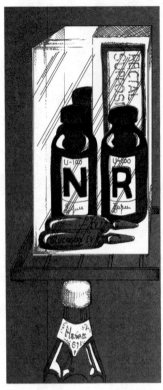

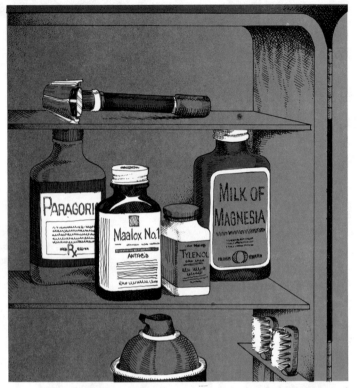

Be prepared
Tell your patient to be prepared
for illness by keeping Paragoric,
Maalox, Tylenol, and Milk of
Magnesia in the medicine cabi-
net and glucagon, rectal sup-
positories, his usual insulin, and
regular insulin in the refrigerator.

dependent diabetic patients but also to those patients on oral
agents if their doctor advises urine tests. The two-drop Clinitest is preferable to the five-drop method because it reduces
the possibility of flashback. (Flashback is the bright orange
color, or 5%, that appears during the boiling process. After
15 seconds, the test will show 2% or 3%. Since this happens
so quickly, the patient often overlooks it, not realizing he
should record the results as 5%.) If directed, the patient should
monitor blood glucose levels (see guidelines on page 80).

● *Take liquids every hour*. Tell the patient to keep a record
of all food and fluids taken and retained and to report this
information to his doctor. Again, this will help the doctor
make necessary adjustments in type and amount of insulin.

Remind the patient that taking small amounts of liquids
frequently helps replenish the fluid he loses through vomiting,
diarrhea, or fever. Encourage him to take 8 oz of liquids, if
he can. Explain that some of the liquids should be a salty
broth, to replace the sodium he loses through vomiting and
diarrhea. This advice applies to all diabetic patients, whether
their diabetes is controlled by diet, oral agents, or insulin.

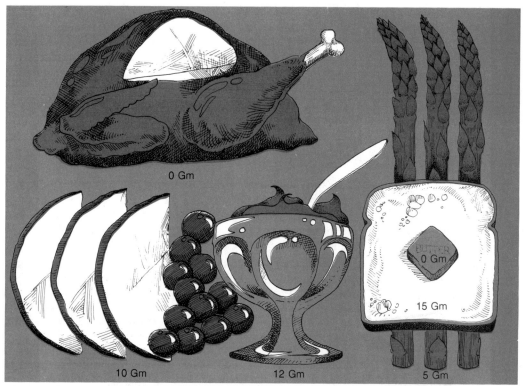

0 Gm

10 Gm

12 Gm

15 Gm

0 Gm

5 Gm

● *If unable to eat the prescribed diet, replace the carbohydrate with liquid or semiliquid foods.* Remind every diabetic patient that carbohydrates are more easily tolerated during illness than proteins or fats and that they affect his blood glucose more rapidly. But if he can't tolerate solid foods, he can replace them with liquid carbohydrates (see page 85).

● *If still unable to eat the prescribed diet after replacing four or five meals with liquid or semiliquid carbohydrates, call the doctor.* Explain to your patient that his diet must be adjusted to include proteins and fats so he can maintain adequate nutrition. Teach him how to calculate replacements for his diet so his insulin dose will be balanced with food.

Applying the guidelines
Now let's see how these guidelines would have applied to Mrs. Armstrong. After taking her morning insulin, she could have asked Mrs. Ryan to stay with her until her husband came home from work. Then she could have gone to bed and kept warm, taking frequent sips of tap water throughout the morning.

At lunch time, Mrs. Ryan could have helped Mrs. Arm-

A healthy lunch for Mrs. Armstrong
When feeling well, Mrs. Armstrong has for lunch three lean meat exchanges, one fruit, one milk (yogurt), one bread, one fat, and one nonstarchy vegetable exchange (about three asparagus spears), amounting to 42 g of carbohydrate.

strong test her urine. The results probably would have been negative for glucose and acetone. She could have replaced the carbohydrate in her prescribed diet with ginger ale, calculating her meal as shown on page 87.

Since ½ cup of ginger ale provides 10 g of carbohydrate, Mrs. Armstrong would have taken 2 cups (40 g). She also could have used the replacement system for her evening meal. She could have taken some bouillon at intervals to replace the sodium she had lost through vomiting, thus maintaining an electrolyte balance. By the following day, she probably would have been able to resume her prescribed diet.

Simple guidelines like these, plus thorough teaching, can help patients maintain control of their diabetes during a short-term illness. But be sure they understand that *no* guidelines can take the place of professional medical care — only a doctor can provide this service. Common sense should guide your patients in deciding which course to follow.

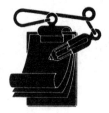

Remember these important points about explaining axioms for sick days to diabetic patients:

1. Help your patient distinguish between short-term illness (persisting less than 48 hours) and long-term illness (persisting longer than 48 hours).

2. Advise a patient with a short-term illness to go to bed and keep warm, test urine glucose levels at least four times a day (or perform blood glucose self-monitoring), take liquids every hour, and continue his insulin regimen.

3. Urge your patient to see a doctor if he has a long-term illness.

4. Stress that not eating or taking insulin may cause diabetic ketoacidosis.

5. Encourage a patient unable to eat the prescribed diet to try substituting liquid or semiliquid foods for carbohydrates.

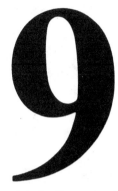

9

Advising the peripatetic diabetic

BY CATHERINE GAROFANO, RN, BS

HELPING PATIENTS MANAGE their diabetes at home involves setting up a routine. But what happens to that routine when a diabetic patient goes on a trip? Very simply, he takes the routine with him. Since this may pose problems, he'll need to do some preplanning and take certain precautions. Here's how you can help.

Planning ahead

First, if your patient doesn't already have some type of medical identification, urge him to get a card or tag identifying him as a diabetic patient and to carry it with him at all times. This identification should include his doctor's name and address and the type and amount of insulin or oral agent he's currently taking.

To ensure that his trip begins without any hitches, suggest that he have a general checkup before leaving. An ordinary but undetected health problem, such as an abscessed tooth, could become particularly traumatic for a diabetic patient in unfamiliar surroundings.

If your patient needs vaccinations or immunizations, tell him to get them a few weeks earlier than usual, since any reactions could affect his diabetes' equilibrium. Of course, if this happens while he's still at home, his own doctor is

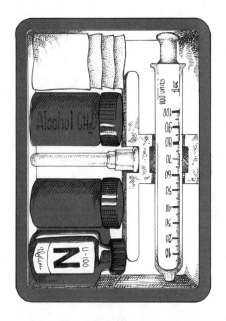

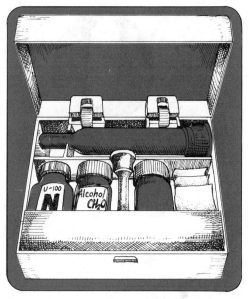

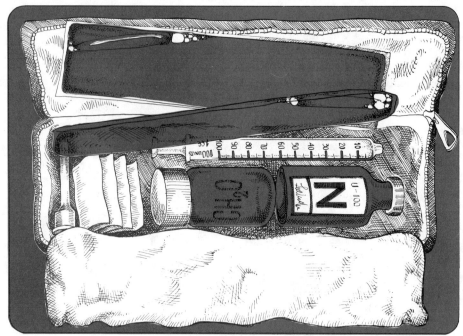

readily available to handle the situation. And having the reaction under control will ease the patient's mind when he sets out on his trip.

You might also suggest that he ask the doctor to prescribe an antidiarrheal agent that he can obtain before leaving. Again, diarrhea is disabling for people without chronic disease; think of the consequences for a diabetic patient!

Of course, you should advise your patient to take along enough medication to last him throughout the trip (although he can obtain foreign equivalents if necessary), as well as syringes, glucagon, and blood or urine testing equipment. Either disposable needles and syringes or a compact kit that includes a reusable syringe, needles, cotton, and a 1-week supply of insulin is convenient for traveling.

If your patient does plan to take along standard syringes, remind him that sterilizing them could be a problem. My patients have reported that hotel kitchens aren't always prepared to give this kind of service.

Suggest that your patient get a written statement from his doctor explaining that he has diabetes and takes insulin by injection. This, along with his medical identification, will facilitate getting syringes through customs as well as getting replacement syringes in a foreign pharmacy, if that should become necessary. (My patients, who've taken these precautions, have traveled to Europe, the Middle East, and the Caribbean without any difficulties going through customs. Diabetes is an international disease, and patients have found that most customs agents recognize medical identification tags and don't question possession of syringes and needles.)

Also, suggest that your patient ask his doctor for a list of his medications by generic name, in case he needs to obtain some in a foreign country. And, as another emergency precaution, if the patient is taking NPH or Lente insulin, suggest that he take a supply of regular insulin along as well.

If your patient is traveling where foreign languages are spoken, emphasize that he learn to say (or carry written messages for) such emergency phrases as: "I am diabetic." "I need a doctor." "May I have a glass of Coca-Cola."

For information about diabetes associations and diabetic care in foreign countries, tell your patient to write to: The International Diabetes Foundation, 3-6 Alfred Place, London, WCIE 7EE, England.

Travel kits for diabetic patients
On the opposite page are three sample travel kits in which diabetic patients can carry their insulin, syringes, alcohol, and cotton swabs. The model on the top left is manufactured by Becton, Dickinson and Company (B-D) of Rutherford, N.J., and is made of inexpensive styrofoam, which helps maintain a cold temperature. On the top right is a more expensive compact B-D kit made of plastic. This kit is not insulated and must be refrigerated to keep insulin cold. The bottom kit, an insulated plastic soft pack made by Graham-Field of New Hyde, N.Y., provides room for all a diabetic patient's needs as well as two freezer packs.

Foreign Equivalents of Oral Hypoglycemics

Orinase (tolbutamide)		Diabinese (chlorpropamide)		Glucotrol (glipizide)	
Canada	Mobenol, Rastinon, Orinase	Denmark	Mellinese	Belgium, Denmark, Germany, Netherlands, Switzerland	Glibenese
Europe	Rastinon, Artosin	Germany	Chloronase, Diabetoral		
France	Dolitol	Italy	Catanil	Spain	Minodiab
Israel	Orsinon	Spain	Chlorodiabet		
Japan	Diabin, Mellitus D	**Dymelor (acetohexamide)**		**Diabeta, Micronase (glyburide)**	
		Chile	Ordimel	Argentina	Pira
Mexico	Yosulant	England	Dimelor	Belgium, Denmark, Netherlands, Norway	Daonil
Philippines	Oralin	Japan	Dimelin		
		Netherlands	Ordimel		
		Norway	Ordimel	Canada	Euglucon
Tolinase (tolazamide)		Sweden	Ordimel	France	Euglucon
Denmark	Orabetta			Hungary	Gilemal
England	Tolanase			Italy	Adiab Gliben
Germany	Norglycin				
Iceland	Tolisan			Spain	Glidiabet Glucolon

Traveling with insulin

Most diabetic patients are concerned about the stability of their insulin while traveling. They want to know: How long will it be stable outside a refrigerator? When will it start to deteriorate? How will extreme temperatures affect it?

Actually, insulin doesn't have to be kept in a refrigerator, but it should be kept in a cool place. For example, tell your patient not to leave insulin in the glove compartment or trunk of a car out in the hot sun all day. But tell him he *can* carry insulin safely in a handbag or briefcase, or in a suitcase between layers of clothing. If he's flying, emphasize that he should carry insulin *with* him rather than leave it in his luggage, since luggage can get lost or delayed.

Assure your patient that all insulins remain stable for months at temperatures of 68° to 75° F. (20° to 23.9° C.). Specifically, NPH, PZI, and Lente insulins remain stable at room temperature for at least 24 months. Neutral regular insulin (NRI) remains stable at room temperature for 18 months, but acid regular insulin (ARI) may lose up to 25% of its potency at room temperature in 6 months. Insulin stability in temperatures ranging from 75° to 100° F. (23.9° to 37.8° C.) hasn't been studied, but at 100° F., all insulins lose a significant amount of potency within 1 to 2 months.

Traveling across time zones

Crossing time zones rapidly, as on a jet flight, requires some adjustment in the diabetes management routine. To make the adjustment as smooth as possible, recommend that your patient request a diabetic diet when he makes his flight reservation. And, since eating on time is important, tell him to identify himself as a diabetic patient to the flight attendants on boarding. If he explains that he must eat at a certain time, they should be able to accommodate him. Of course, he should always carry snacks — for example, peanut butter crackers or hard candy — in case of a delay.

Adjusting insulin dosage also requires planning. You can help your patient make his adjustment by giving him these tips:

- Take your usual dose of NPH or Lente insulin, with or without regular insulin.
- Keep your watch set according to departure time.
- If more than 24 hours have elapsed when you arrive at your destination (for example, if you've traveled from east to west), take a small amount of regular or intermediate insulin to cover the additional hours gained, *unless* your voided urine specimen is negative or your blood sugar (as determined by self-monitoring) is within the normal range. (Consult your doctor beforehand about the exact amount of additional insulin to take.)
- If less than 24 hours have elapsed when you arrive, take less insulin the following morning. (Again, your doctor will tell you how much less.)
- After taking insulin in the new time zone, set your watch according to the new time.
- The following day, take your usual dose of insulin.
- Follow the same plan (in reverse) on the return trip.

As an extra precaution, recommend that your patient take an antinauseant at least 4 hours before departure time. If he becomes ill despite this precaution, suggest that he take an antiemetic suppository.

If your patient plans to drive extensively, advise him to take 10 g of carbohydrate every hour (for example, an orange, peach, or pear; two graham crackers; or three Life Savers) and to stop frequently and walk around. And, again, suggest that he carry extra snacks in case of a breakdown or delay.

Adjusting activities

The diabetic traveler must adjust his activities to his manage-

Have language, will travel

When traveling in foreign countries, a diabetic patient should learn to say or have written down: "I am diabetic." "Please get me a doctor." "Sugar or Coca-Cola, please."

I am diabetic.
French: "Je suis diabétique."
Spanish: "Yo soy diabético."
German: "Ich bin zuckerkrank."
Italian: "Io sono diabetico."

Please get me a doctor.
French: "Allez chercher un médecin, s'il vous plait."
Spanish: "Haga me el favor de llamar al médico."
German: "Rufen sie bitte einen Arzt."
Italian: 'Per favore chiami un dottore."

Sugar or Coca-Cola, please.
French: "Sucre ou Coca-Cola, s'il vous plait."
Spanish: "Azúcar o un vaso de Coca-Cola, por favor."
German: "Zucker oder Coca-Cola, bitte."
Italian: "Succhero o Coca-Cola, per favore."

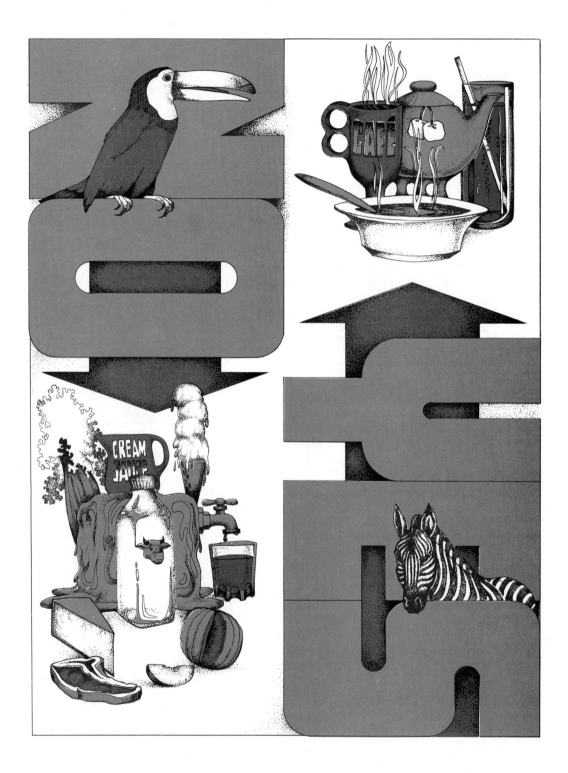

ment routine, too. Urge him to keep up with his regular amount of exercise, but warn him not to overexert himself. Stress that before participating in any strenuous activity or exercise — even sight-seeing — he should either decrease his morning insulin dose by 10% or eat extra carbohydrate (fruit, crackers, or milk).

If he's going skiing, caution him against wearing boots that are too tight around his ankles or legs, since they will impair circulation. If he's going to a beach, remind him never to walk barefoot, even on sand. Advise him to wear sandles to protect his feet against cuts. Remind him, too, to limit the time he spends in the hot sun and to always protect himself against sunburn by applying a screening lotion.

If your patient anticipates doing a lot of walking, he should, of course, wear comfortable shoes. Remind him that even shoes he's worn before can cause problems after walking in them for several hours. Suggest that he pay extra attention to proper foot care. If he develops blisters, warn him not to open them nor to apply adhesive tape directly to his skin. If he must apply Band-Aids, recommend that he use those that have Telfa-coated pads.

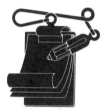

Remember these important points about advising the peripatetic diabetic:
1. Urge your patient to wear Medic Alert jewelry or carry a card identifying him as diabetic at all times.
2. Suggest that he have a general checkup before leaving on a trip and get any vaccinations a few weeks earlier than customary.
3. To get syringes through customs, advise him to obtain a written statement from his doctor explaining that he's diabetic and takes insulin by injection.
4. Have your patient ask his doctor for a list of his medications by generic name, in case he needs to obtain them in a foreign country.
5. Teach your patient how to adjust his insulin dosage when traveling across time zones.

S₂KILLCHECK

1. Frank Melton, age 67, takes 36 units of Semilente insulin every morning. When he brings in his Clinitest results from the previous week, they look like this:

	DAY 1	DAY 2	DAY 3	DAY 4	DAY 5	DAY 6	DAY 7
Before breakfast	2	3	4	3	4	3	4
Before lunch	2	1	2	1	1	1	1
Before dinner	Trace	0	1	Trace	0	Trace	Trace
Before bedtime snack	3	4	4	3	3	3	3

How would you advise him to change his therapy?

2. Gretchen Hanson, age 17, has been taking 30 units of U-100 Semilente insulin every morning for about 2 months. At first she controlled her diabetes well. But now she says that she's getting a variable response to therapy. You ask her to describe her injection techniques. She says she always makes sure she's using a U-100 syringe with her U-100 insulin. Then she shakes the bottle to mix the insulin, wipes the top with an alcohol swab, pulls the plunger out to 30, removes the needle cover, and inserts the needle into the bottle top. She pushes the plunger in, inverts the bottle, pulls the plunger back to 30 units, and withdraws the needle from the bottle. Then she inserts the ½" needle straight into the injection site, checks for blood, and injects the insulin if the needle isn't in a vein. She says, too, that she's very conscientious about rotating injection sites. What is Gretchen doing wrong?

3. Bill Preston, a diabetic patient who takes 8 units of regular insulin and 32 units of NPH insulin every morning, is being sent on a 1-week business trip to Paris. His plane leaves at noon Eastern Standard Time (EST) and arrives at 1:20 a.m. Paris time (early evening EST). Mr. Preston plans to go

directly to his hotel from the airport, check in for the night, and get up early the next morning (3 a.m. EST). A week later he'll return on an early morning flight (1:10 a.m. EST) that will arrive home at 10:20 a.m. EST. What adjustments should he make in therapy to account for the change in time zones?

4. Jill Collins has an upset stomach with some diarrhea. She calls you in the afternoon asking what she should do about her therapy. She says she took her usual 500 mg of Orinase this morning but, since she doesn't feel like eating, she wonders if she should skip her pill tomorrow. What's your advice?

5. Fifteen-year-old Pat, a Type I diabetic, has had difficulty keeping her diabetes under strict control. But this week she proudly announces that during the past 2 days her urine tests have read negative before breakfast, at lunch, before dinner, and even at bedtime. What would you tell her?

6. Randy Thomas tells you he's been feeling tired, thirsty, and flushed for the past few afternoons. He says he's taking the right amount of Semilente and Lente insulins and sticking to his dietary therapy, so he can't understand why he feels that way. Because the feeling usually disappears in the early evening, though, he says he's not worried about it. What would you expect Randy's urine tests to show? Would you advise Randy to make any changes in his diabetic therapy?

7. Marvin Kissinger is retiring this year after 40 years of service at his company. As a retirement gift, the company is fulfilling Marvin's lifelong dream — a trip to Germany to visit the cousins he has never met. Marvin was just recently diagnosed as a diabetic. Fortunately, he can control his diabetes with diet alone. But he wonders if he should make any special arrangements for the trip because of his diabetes. What would you tell him?

(Answers begin on page 205)

HOW TO COPE
WITH COMPLICATIONS

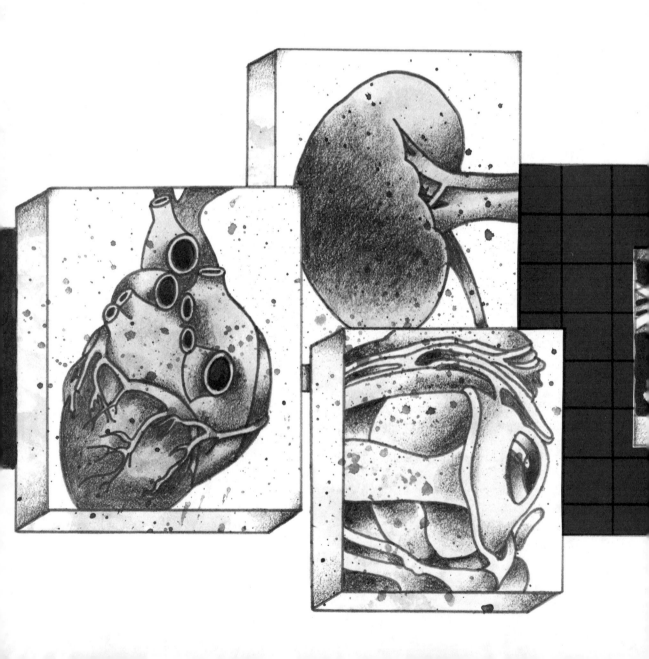

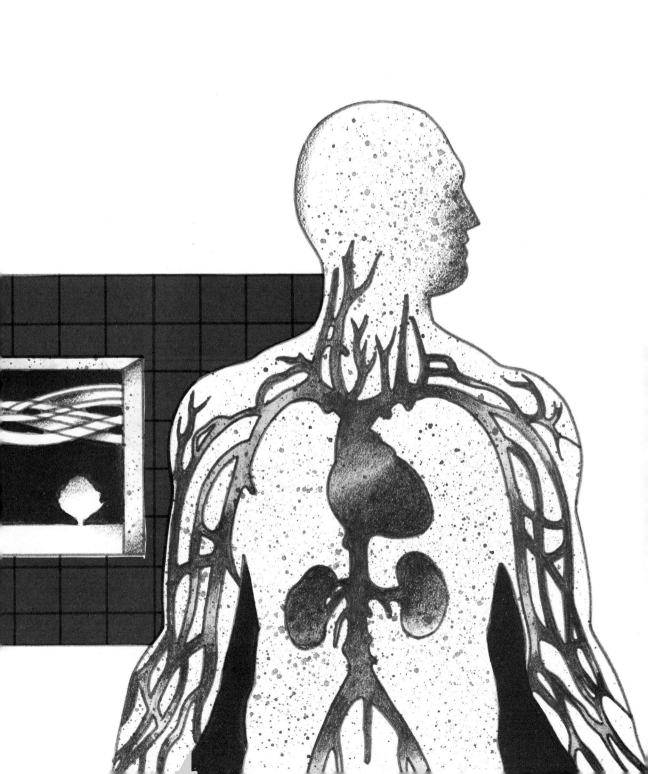

What eye abnormalities would you expect to find during your assessment of a diabetic patient?

What precipitates symptoms of hypoglycemia?

If your patient has insulin-induced hypoglycemia, what initial care would you give to stabilize his blood glucose level?

When treating diabetic ketoacidosis (DKA), what is the best way to calculate insulin dosage?

How does hyperglycemic hyperosmolar nonketotic coma (HHNC) differ from DKA and other hyperglycemia-related conditions?

10

Mastering the art of assessment

BY DELORES SCHUMANN, RN, MS, FAAN

CATARACTS; CARDIOVASCULAR disease; kidney failure; neuropathies of the bladder, eyes, GI tract, hands and feet, and reproductive system; periodontal disease; peripheral vascular disorders; retinopathy; skin lesions and infections; urinary tract infections.... Sound like an excerpt from an index of diseases? It's not. It's a list of *some* of the complications of diabetes mellitus...complications you may be able to help prevent.

The first step to preventive health care for a diabetic patient is physical assessment. Which of the many possible ills afflict him? How can he avoid the others? What are the signs and symptoms to look for? How do you answer the questions — some spoken and some unspoken — that worry him? How, in brief, can you make your best contribution to the difficult art of managing a patient with diabetes?

Your physical assessment can begin the moment you meet the patient. Note his general appearance and behavior, his clothing and his gait — these can be your first clues to his sensory and motor status. If you shake hands with him, look for atrophy of his hand muscles, an indication of neurologic impairment.

Here are other things to examine:

Dermopathy

1. *Shin spots* may be caused by trauma.
2. In about 15% of patients, *necrobiosis lipoidica diabeticorum* precedes onset of diabetes by 2 years.
3. *Pyoderma with ulceration* can develop when minor infections are not treated.
4. *Tuberous xanthomas* appear on the buttocks, knees, and elbows; when lipids return to normal level, the xanthomas disappear.

The skin

As you know, the diabetic patient is easy prey to skin infections. Normally, glucose disappears from the skin at a rate of about 2%/minute; in the diabetic patient, the rate has slowed to 0.3%/minute. The resulting glucose pool under the epidermis creates an ideal medium for cutaneous infections, especially in the groin, axillae, and inframammary areas.

Obese women, in particular, are susceptible to the growth of *Candida albicans,* which may result from the high moisture and glucose content of skin-to-skin chafing. So, look for signs of that infection: it makes the skin beefy-red to violet-red. The surface oozes, and small pustular lesions surround the clearly defined infected area.

We recently treated a woman in our clinic whose *Candida* infection of the groin had stubbornly resisted treatment. We persuaded her to substitute cotton pants for nylon ones and to stop sitting for long periods on chairs with plastic-covered seats. That worked: her infection cleared up.

Check the shins of your diabetic patient for brown spots — small brown scars with a shallow depression. The brownish color is believed to come from iron-containing substances that remain after small internal hemorrhages. The shin is subject to more trauma than most other areas of the body; and therefore, the brown spots. The brown spots are harmless, but they are a clue to widespread blood vessel changes in the diabetic patient.

Look also for necrobiosis lipoidica diabeticorum, another lesion seen on the shin; it also results from small vessel disease. It's reddish-yellow and atrophic, and progresses until it covers a large area of the skin of the lower anterior legs. Despite its appearance, it is harmless.

Watch for pinkish-yellow papules over elbows and knees (xanthomas). They indicate grossly elevated blood fats, especially triglycerides. Although these are not limited to diabetic patients, they call attention to the continued need for assessing blood fats.

Look especially for skin lesions caused by insulin injection. Fatty accumulation beneath the skin, similar to a lipoma, may form with repeated injection. Patients prefer to use these sites because they tend to become fibrous and insensitive to needle puncture, but insulin will be absorbed poorly from such sites. If you see that your patient needs excessive amounts of insulin

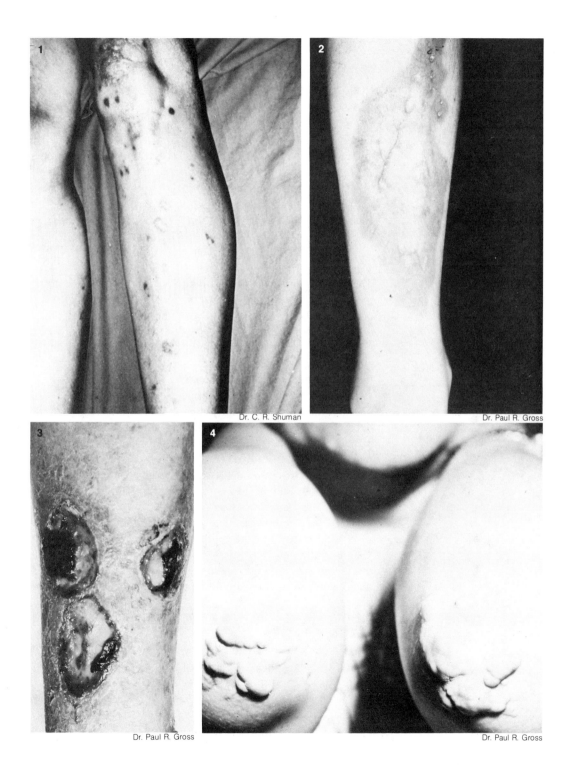

Dr. C. R. Shuman

Dr. Paul R. Gross

Dr. Paul R. Gross

Dr. Paul R. Gross

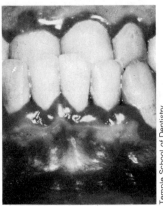

Temple School of Dentistry

Control the diabetes first
In diabetic patients, some conditions won't respond to treatment until the diabetes itself is brought under control. This patient had refractory subacute gingivitis. Since his condition did not respond to therapy, his doctors suspected that he might have diabetes. Once the doctors stabilized his blood glucose level with insulin, they were at last able to cure the gingivitis.

to keep his diabetes under control, examine his injection sites to see if they have undergone fatty degeneration.

You may see atrophic areas at the injection sites. Patients are more distressed by these because of their hollowed-out appearance. They, too, are harmless and can be prevented by rotating and distributing injection sites. If the patient has scars at injection sites, suspect improper injection technique — insulin is given subcutaneously at a 45° to 90° angle. When insulin is injected superficially — that is, intradermally — a wheal raises with each injection. Then scarring follows, as after a smallpox vaccination.

The mouth
The diabetic patient is susceptible to periodontal disease, commonly called pyorrhea. It eventually destroys the bony supporting structures of the tooth, and the tooth loosens or falls out. Periodontal disease does not always appear as an obvious swelling and bleeding of the gums; sometimes, it goes undetected until the dentist finds substantial bone loss from around the teeth when he probes or looks at the dental X-rays.

Poor oral hygiene and accumulation of dental plaque invite periodontal disease. Dental plaque is a mix of bacteria, food debris, and dead cells deposited from a microscopic layer of protein (called the pellicle) that normally coats all tooth surfaces. If plaque is allowed to accumulate, it hardens, becomes calculus, and then provides a nesting ground for more bacteria.

Teach your patient how to remove this dental plaque daily. He must use dental floss to remove the plaque from spaces between the teeth where the toothbrush doesn't reach, also using proper brushing technique up and down. Plaque is invisible to the naked eye; to see it, the patient must dissolve a disclosing tablet in his mouth to stain the plaque red. His dental care, of course, should be closely supervised by a dentist.

The eyes
The patient's vision should be assessed by recording his visual acuity at each clinic visit and by making a funduscopic examination every 6 months.

He can develop a variety of visual problems. Early in his disease, the diabetic patient may notice blurred vision, prompting him to ask to have his glasses changed. This blurring may result from fluctuations in glucose levels which distort the lens of the eye. With high blood glucose levels, sorbitol and fructose accumulate in the lens; the lens swells and distorts vision. As blood glucose subsides to normal levels, the lens returns to its original shape, and vision may improve. That is why the patient should wait 6 to 8 weeks after his treatment begins before obtaining new glasses.

Accumulation of fructose and sorbitol can also cause cataracts. The lens swells, fibers deteriorate, and the clefts between the fibers fill up with a proteinaceous substance. The lens becomes milky white and opaque. With the light from a flashlight, you can see the opacity as gray against the black pupil. With the ophthalmoscope, you can see the opacity as gray or black against the red reflex.

Although no one's proved it, chronic simple glaucoma seems to be especially prevalent in the diabetic patient. Ask your patient whether he has frequent headaches, sees halos around lights, or has impaired peripheral vision, evidenced by colliding with furniture or, when attempting to cross the street, narrowly avoiding an oncoming car. Look for further clues: a red conjunctiva or a pupil unresponsive to light (fixed in size). Palpate the globe: A hard consistency suggests increased intraocular tension and glaucoma. Peripheral vision can be estimated with the visual confrontation test. The best check for glaucoma, of course, is with the tonometer. When visual abnormalities are suspected, a thorough evaluation should be made by an ophthalmologist.

Retinopathy is by far the most *common* eye problem for the diabetic patient. Diabetic retinopathy consists of microaneurysms (outpouchings or balloonlike structures on the walls of small retinal vessels) and neovascularization. The new vessels are weak and poorly supported. Serum and blood leak from them because they are so fragile. If a patient has a small hemorrhage from one of these vessels, he may notice "little dark streaks" in his vision. A large area of bleeding appears to him as a red film that blocks his vision completely. These hemorrhages can destroy vision. They may involve not only the retina; they can also rupture into the vitreous. They require a long time for absorption — if they are large enough, they may not be absorbed at all — and scarring follows. The result is markedly impaired vision or blindness.

With the funduscope, check the entire retina, because the

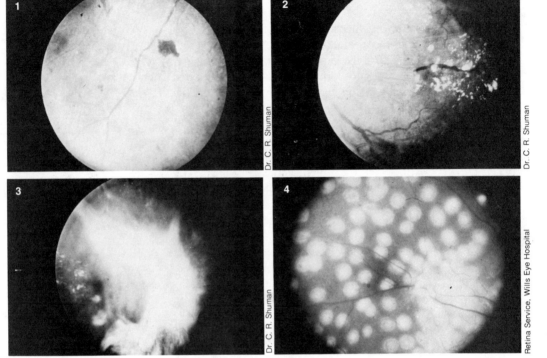

Retinopathy

1. *Microaneurysms and hemorrhage* appear as the earliest changes in retinal blood vessels.
2. *Hard exudates, fresh preretinal hemorrhage* (in middle of field), *and neovascularization* appear in the more advanced stages of the disease.
3. With *retinitis proliferans*, the patient is frequently considered legally blind.
4. *Photocoagulation,* in this case with an argon laser, can stop the progress of retinopathy.

changes may differ from one part to another. You may notice soft exudates — "cotton wool spots" — where a retinal artery has become occluded and a soft exuding takes place. You may see rings of fluid or serum around microaneurysms, or yellowish blots (known as hard exudates) where this fluid was absorbed but left behind lipid material. Check carefully for dilatation, tortuosity, or irregularity in the caliber of vessels.

Remember that a patient can have retinopathy without visual impairment, which occurs only when the hemorrhage or the exudate involves the macula.

An ophthalmologist must follow the progress of the diabetic patient who has retinopathy, but you can contribute by making periodic checks of the retina. Although experience is necessary to correctly identify funduscopic features of the diabetic eye, many nurses are acquiring this skill.

The cardiovascular system

Although the diabetic patient, like the general population, invites heart disease with increased blood pressure, obesity, heavy cigarette smoking, and high blood cholesterol, diabetes itself is among the high-risk factors for arteriosclerotic heart disease. But evidence strongly suggests that development of vascular lesions can be halted by careful diabetic control consisting of normal blood glucose levels, normal weight, and normal blood lipid levels.

Check the patient's weight and blood pressure systematically. Discuss with him the importance of weight control and physical fitness. As weight is reduced, elevated cholesterol levels decrease slightly, and triglyceride levels decrease substantially. Physical fitness is believed to help lower triglycerides.

Listen carefully for comments relative to his cardiac status. Does he experience recurrent chest pains, suggesting angina pectoris? Anginal pain is produced by exertion and subsides when the activity ceases. The pain is felt in the chest and sometimes also in the neck, arms, and even the back. Does he take medication for the pain, and to what extent does it relieve the pain? Some patients have chest wall pain not associated with exercise, which produces anxiety because it resembles angina pectoris.

The doctor may request an electrocardiogram. Remember that a high percentage of patients with angina pectoris and no prior myocardial infarction have a normal EKG at rest.

The peripheral vascular system
A patient with peripheral vascular problems often will tell you he has leg pains that begin when he walks and end when he stops (intermittent claudication). If he has an acute obstruction in a vessel, the pain will persist after he stops. Ordinarily, pain starts in the calf, but, depending on the site of occlusion, it can start in the foot, thigh, hip, or buttocks.

Inspect the legs and feet to judge the competence of circulation. In arterial insufficiency, the extremities are pale, but there is no edema. The skin is cool, shiny, atrophic, and thin-appearing. Nails are thick and ridged, and the patient may tell you that they grow more slowly. There is loss of hair over the dorsum of the foot. Note the strength of the pedal pulses; in arterial insufficiency, they are decreased, absent, or *"pipe-stem–like."* Circulatory competence may also be assessed by using the ultrasound stethoscope. Because of the Doppler effect, this device's ultrahigh-frequency sound waves can help you estimate arterial blood flow. Or, check for arterial competency by elevating the patient's legs 30 cm. Ask him to move his feet up and down; then look for blanching and un-

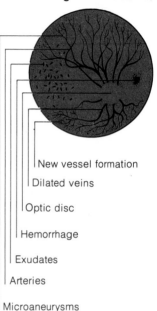

Retinal damage due to diabetes

New vessel formation

Dilated veins

Optic disc

Hemorrhage

Exudates

Arteries

Microaneurysms

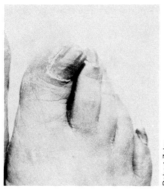

Even toenails are affected
As arterial circulation breaks
down, the diabetic patient's toenails become thick and ridged
and grow more slowly.

usual pallor. After this, have him sit with legs dangling. In about 10 seconds, the normal color should return to his legs; a dusky rubor that develops slowly signals arterial insufficiency.

Inspect the legs and feet for ulcerations. With ischemia from the arterial insufficiency, any trauma to the thin, atrophic skin produces ulcers that heal slowly, become a site for infection, and may lead to gangrene.

For many patients, drugs, such as reserpine, guanethidine, and methyldopa, help relieve peripheral vascular problems. These drugs — which act on the sympathetic nervous system — work to improve cutaneous capillary blood flow.

The kidney and bladder

Kidney disease usually develops gradually. The first signs may be recurring urinary tract infections or albumin (protein), pus cells, or possibly visible blood in the urine. Also watch for changes in laboratory values; for example, increased serum creatinine, BUN, and phosphorus levels; and decreased hemoglobin, hematocrit, calcium, and creatinine clearance levels. Symptoms may be intermittent, or absent.

Even with advanced kidney failure, a patient may offer only vague signs and symptoms: feelings of fatigue, easy exhaustion, muscular weakness, and pallor. Because these symptoms are nonspecific, it may be difficult to decide whether to investigate them. Nevertheless, check to see if the patient has noticed swelling of his ankles or face, increased urination at night, generalized itching, bone pain, easy bleeding, or a peculiar odor to his breath. Remember that only a few of these symptoms may be present in the early phases of kidney failure.

What causes this kidney failure? Diabetes often causes changes in the glomerular capillaries. The basement membrane of the capillaries becomes thick and abnormally porous, allowing protein and red blood cells to pass into the urine. The filtering ability of the kidney is also diminished, allowing waste products to accumulate in the blood.

If the patient is known to have kidney impairment, look for the extent of his edema by checking the pretibial area, the sacrum, ankles and feet, and the conjunctiva. Changes in the kidneys' insulin clearance and insulin metabolism may increase or decrease the patient's insulin needs; check for any evidences of insulin hypoglycemia.

Also review the patient's program for control of the renal

problem. Most often the diet is limited in protein and sodium; vitamins and minerals may be supplemented. Also, he may be taking medication to control blood pressure; review its proper administration with him.

Urinary tract infections are common in patients with neurogenic bladders. The diabetic patient is also prone to a condition called necrotizing papillitis, a result of infection in the renal pyramids associated with vascular disease. Symptoms that occur together in urinary tract infections are frequency and urgency of urination, and dysuria. Besides the symptoms common to urinary tract infections, the patient may have a sudden urge to void and lose urine before he is able to get to the bathroom (urge incontinence). To determine his condition, be sure to question the patient about possible gross hematuria and nocturia.

Bladder infections in the diabetic patient may cause pneumaturia — the production of hydrogen gas when bacteria act upon glucose in bladder urine. The voided urine becomes bubbly. Tell the patient about the significance of bubbly urine and advise him, if it occurs, to contact a doctor immediately. Should you have an occasion to catheterize a diabetic patient with pneumaturia, removal of the urine is followed by an explosive passage of gas. Pneumaturia is a clue to recurrence of bacterial bladder infections.

Neuropathies

Neuropathy in the diabetic patient affects many structures and gives rise to a broad range of clinical manifestations, ranging from extraocular muscle palsies to the more common peripheral nerve problems. As you assess a patient's status, be alert to the various areas it can affect. Pay attention to his upper extremities, particularly his hands. Look for atrophy of the small muscles; this is most marked in the interosseal space between the thumb and first finger. Cigarette burns on the fingers or painless burns on the hands acquired while cooking are clues to the extent of sensory impairment. (Blind diabetic patients have difficulty in mastering braille because of the impaired sensation of touch.)

Dysfunctions of the extraocular muscles are due most often to impairment of cranial nerves three, four, and six, usually three and six. The first thing you might hear from the patient is that he has a severe pain — a headache, a forehead pain,

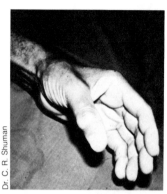

Dr. C. R. Shuman

Neuropathy in the extremities
Patients can suffer atrophy of the interosseous muscle, most marked between the thumb and the index finger. The hands become weak, clumsy, and insensitive to pain. In the feet, neuropathy causes the toes to curl up, pulling the metatarsal pads out of place. As the patient walks, blisters form and, without treatment, can develop into ulcers.

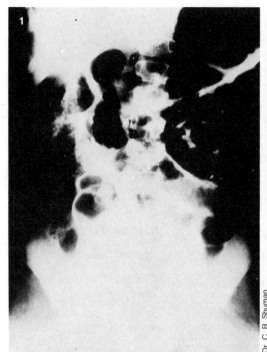
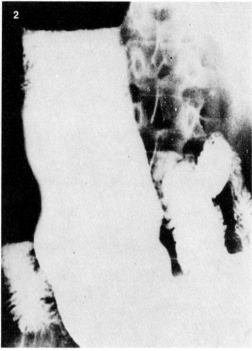

Dr. C. R. Shuman

The not so obvious

1. *Gastrointestinal tract* — Here you will see that the patient's muscle tone has broken down. The emptying of his stomach will be difficult and irregular, impairing control of his diabetes. He may also develop ulcer-like symptoms.

2. *Genitourinary tract* — This diabetic patient's bladder is severely distended and atonic. As his sensory nerves break down, the autonomic reflex to urinate also deteriorates and he will have trouble voiding, greatly increasing the chance of secondary infection.

or an eye pain — on the affected side. Later, he develops double vision. Examine the range of the extraocular movements to identify the paresis. Pupil function is not affected. Symptoms disappear spontaneously without treatment.

Gastrointestinal (GI) tract. Neuropathy affecting the GI tract gives rise to delayed gastric emptying, symptoms suggesting malabsorption of food, and diarrhea, among others. The diarrhea occurs often enough to merit further attention. Patients complain about intermittent, unpredictable diarrheal attacks that vary in length. They may have alternating periods of constipation and diarrhea. During a diarrheal episode, the stools are most frequent in the late evening, at night, and in the early morning. Stools are brown and watery. Abdominal distress and painful straining do not accompany the diarrhea. Your patient may be embarrassed to discuss his symptoms because of nocturnal fecal incontinence.

Bladder dysfunction. A diabetic is susceptible to neurogenic bladder, often leading to infection, interference with urination, and painless retention of urine in the bladder. He may first notice a bladder problem because of infrequent voiding — perhaps only once or twice a day. He may have a weak stream or dribbling, or he may strain to void the urine. Symptoms can go unrecognized until the abdomen increases in size, suggesting a tumor. A patient may seek medical help because he has symptoms of a bladder infection but is unaware of the actual problem. (Males may actually have prostatic hypertrophy.)

Reproductive function. Both male and female diabetic patients experience sexual dysfunction. Although authorities disagree on the etiology of impotence in diabetic men, most believe it is neurogenic. About 50% of diabetic men have organic impotence. They usually retain normal sexual interest, but they notice a slow onset of erectile dysfunction — described as 50% firm. Masturbation is ineffective in attaining an erection.

What is thought to be the cause? Nerve impairment impedes the transfer of the impulse that causes the penile arteries to dilate, hindering engorgement of blood that is necessary for an erection. This impotence is irreversible; administration of testosterone does not help.

The patient may also experience retrograde ejaculation. He has an orgasm, but there is no ejaculate. Incompetence of the bladder neck allows the seminal fluid to flow back into the bladder instead of being propelled to the outside. Until recently, there was little medical help for this problem. In 1974, one group of researchers used phenylpropanolamine (Ornade) for a diabetic patient with retrograde ejaculation. Semen volume immediately increased, and ejaculation occurred. Following 2 months of treatment, the sperm count, motility, and morphology were normal.

Any male diabetic patient who seeks help with fertility and sterility problems needs careful examination and counseling to determine whether diabetic impotence is the cause of the problem. Although there is no cure if the impotence arises from diabetic neuropathy, sound explanations to the patient and his spouse can alleviate many anxieties and correct misinformation. When impotence lacks an organic cause, counseling may include referring the patient to a urologist for possible penile implant surgery.

Information about sexual dysfunction in the diabetic female patient is scanty. Orgasmic difficulties do occur, developing gradually over a period of 6 months to 1 year after the onset of diabetes mellitus.

Peripheral neuropathy. Peripheral neuropathy affects all extremities, most often the feet and legs. It is bilateral and symmetrical. The patient often is bewildered because he has

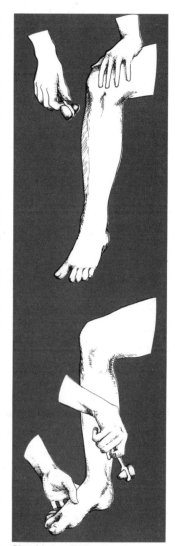

Checking reflexes
To pick up early neuropathy in diabetic patients, routinely check knee and ankle jerks. With the patient sitting with knees flexed, tap the patellar tendon. Note quadriceps contraction. Dorsiflex the ankle with patient's leg flexed. Tap the Achilles' tendon; watch for plantar flexion of the ankle.

Watch your step!
Diabetic patients can lose the arch in the *Charcot's joint:* the bones collapse on themselves (photo 1, on opposite page). Note the contrast with the normal foot on the right. Because of neuropathies and circulatory impairment, lesions and sepsis also can lead to many serious foot problems, such as gangrene (photo 2) and ischemic ulcers (photos 3 and 4).

pain in his legs at night but not during the day. He may tell you that the pain is not apparent until nighttime; it may not even be present when he goes to bed, but it awakens him during the night. It may disappear again early in the morning. It is relieved by walking. (Remember, pain from arterial insufficiency is intensified by walking.) Question him carefully about paresthesia. Burning, numbness, tingling, itching, or a feeling of walking on cotton or pillows are common. Be alert to the effects of decreased sensation to *high or low* temperature. The patient may have erythematous, blistered, or ulcerated areas because he has used excessive heat to warm his legs and feet. Examine the deep tendon reflexes; in peripheral neuropathy of diabetes, the ankle jerks may be absent.

Lack of sensation in the extremities can lead to bizarre results. A young married woman showed up at our clinic with dozens of peculiar red spots on her hands and forearms. She was being treated for her diabetes. What was this new problem? Skin infection? Rash? Drug reaction? Detective work revealed that she cooked fried eggs for her husband nearly every morning, and never felt the tiny burns she received from spattering grease.

The diabetic foot
Examination of a diabetic patient is incomplete until you have thoroughly examined the feet and interdigital spaces and have felt the pedal pulses. Neuropathy affects the diabetic foot by causing changes either in the muscle or in the bony structures. The result of the muscular changes is that the toes become ''cocked up'' or assume a clawing position. This exposes the metatarsal heads. The patient adjusts his gait to the new toe position, forcing foot areas not ordinarily accustomed to the stress of walking to assume it. Calluses form at the metatarsal heads and at sites of walking pressure. Eventually, ulcers develop over these areas.

The result of the bony structure changes is loss of sensation around the joint and relaxation of the supporting tissues. The joint is not buffered as the patient walks, and eventually it becomes jammed. There is swelling but no fluid accumulation. The foot becomes shorter and wider, and the longitudinal arch is completely flattened — it may have a ''rocker-bottom'' appearance. As a result, the patient develops an abnormal gait to compensate for this, again allowing new pressure

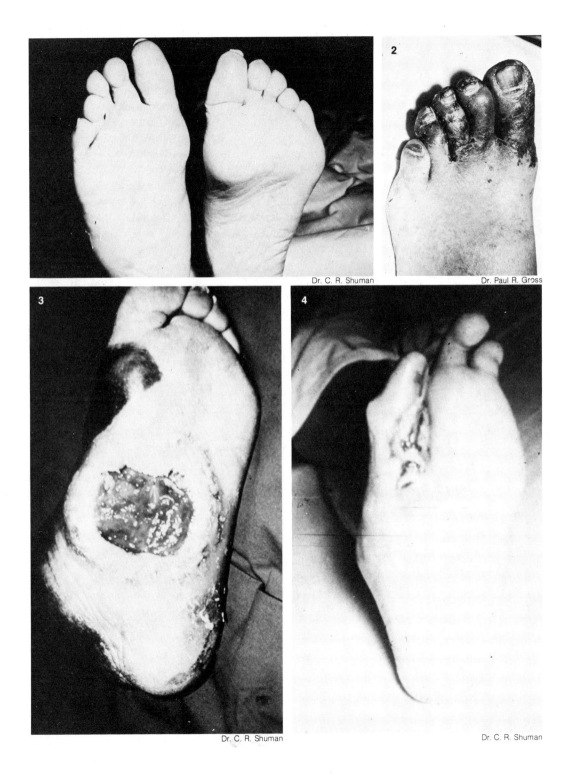

Dr. C. R. Shuman

Dr. Paul R. Gross

Dr. C. R. Shuman

Dr. C. R. Shuman

points and ulcers to develop.

As you inspect the feet, look carefully for neuropathic ulcers. They are usually painless and occur at sites of pressure. Do not neglect the soles of the feet, for the patient may be unaware that an object in his shoe is creating a pressure area. One of our patients developed an ulcer on the bottom of his foot because the heads of two nails protruded on the inside of his shoe. He was oblivious to the ulcer and the nails.

Inspect the feet for calluses. These result from abnormal pressure on the foot, usually from ill-fitting shoes. Once better-fitting shoes are worn, calluses gradually disappear. You can teach your diabetic patient to use an emery board or pumice stone to remove the roughened aspects of the calluses. Trimming calluses to remove the hard keratin and expose the soft keratin should be done by a qualified person, such as a podiatrist, physician, or nurse.

Examine the skin of the feet and the nails for evidences of infection. Thick, yellow nails may indicate a fungus infection. Discoloration starts at the open end of the nail and spreads to the nail root. Eventually, the nail begins to separate from the toe and becomes crumbly.

Remember these important points about assessing a diabetic patient for complications:
1. Inspect the skin for shin spots, necrobiosis lipoidica diabeticorum, pyoderma with ulceration, and tuberous xanthomas.
2. Check the mouth for signs of periodontal disease.
3. Examine the eyes for cataracts, glaucoma, and retinopathy.
4. Use an ultrasound stethoscope to estimate arterial blood flow in a patient with peripheral vascular problems.
5. If your patient has kidney disease, watch for laboratory value changes, such as increased serum creatinine, BUN, and phosphorus levels; and decreased hemoglobin, hematocrit, calcium, and creatinine clearance levels.

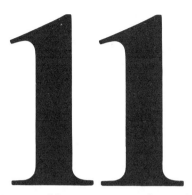

11

Insulin reactions:
Fighting fear and fact

BY DELORES SCHUMANN, RN, MS, FAAN

PATIENTS AND health-care providers fear insulin reactions — with good reason. Damage from severe, repeated, and prolonged hypoglycemia can lead to ischemic necrosis of the brain, notably of the vasomotor center. Irreversible damage to neurons can impair intellectual ability and lead to personality changes. In patients with atherosclerosis, insulin reaction may lead to myocardial infarction as well. Retinal hemorrhages commonly appear after an attack.

And yet these are admittedly extremes. For most persons with diabetes, the *fear* of a reaction will fortunately continue to be worse than the reaction itself or its aftereffects. Perhaps the fear shouldn't be dispelled at that. Perhaps it can help you teach the person with diabetes to concentrate on preventing hypoglycemia. In fact, some diabetologists purposely induce a mild reaction so the patient can experience one under safe, controlled conditions.

Abnormally low blood glucose levels can result from causes other than injected insulin. Other possible causes include:

- *severe liver disease,* which greatly reduces glycogen uptake and release from the liver

- *adrenocortical insufficiency,* in which the leading glucocorticoids (cortisol and cortisone) aren't present to stimulate gluconeogenesis (the process whereby the liver forms carbo-

Elusive hypoglycemia
Of the people who have hypoglycemic episodes, more than
half experience no warning
symptoms. So when teaching
patients, stress the importance
of testing for glucose in their
blood or urine on a regular basis.

hydrates from proteins and fats)

• *islet cell tumor*, which uses up available glucose by over-producing insulin.

Blood glucose can drop, too, when *oral* drugs are used to control diabetes, or when some potentiating drug is given in combination with an oral antidiabetic agent. But here, let's deal only with hypoglycemia from insulin injection.

Not every patient knows

Most diabetic patients are aware of an oncoming hypoglycemic reaction and can take steps to reverse it. *But a significant number do not recognize premonitory symptoms, and some simply do not display the symptoms.*

Much of our patient education has been geared to the first group, who have an intact sympathetic response, do have symptoms, do recognize them, and do ward off the insulin reaction with food. Even then, too little food or more exercise than usual may alter their response.

For example, after a hard week's work at the office, Betty S., age 32, arose one Saturday, took her 40 units of Semilente insulin, ate her usual breakfast, and went off with friends for a morning of tennis. By 1 o'clock, as they returned home, she seemed a little vague and was yawning. Her well-meaning guests, thinking this ordinary fatigue, urged her to take a nap while they prepared lunch. Her husband recognized what was happening and insisted that she drink 4 oz of orange juice. Shortly, she felt nearly normal again.

Her doctor explained that exercise potentiates insulin. So, when she plays weekend tennis now, Mrs. S. cuts her daily dose of insulin (and is not afraid to eat some of her usual emergency supply of hard candy).

Among a second group of puzzling patients are many older people with diabetes who (especially if they have cerebral arteriosclerosis) experience the usual sympathetic response and show the usual symptoms, but seem never to comprehend their meaning. Probably their cerebral function is compromised. Now a slight decline in blood glucose further impairs their ability to reason or recognize their symptoms, let alone cope with them. By the time the bodily adrenergic response releases epinephrine, they are too confused to act on it.

Much of our educational effort should surely aim at trying to make these patients more alert to their own situation. And

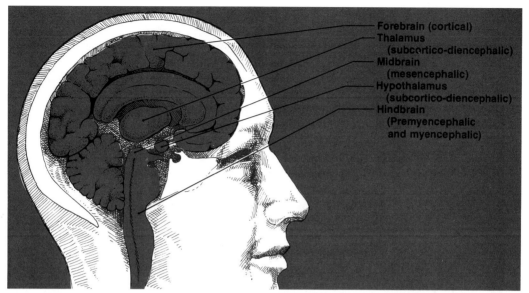

Forebrain (cortical)
Thalamus
 (subcortico-diencephalic)
Midbrain
 (mesencephalic)
Hypothalamus
 (subcortico-diencephalic)
Hindbrain
 (Premyencephalic
 and myencephalic)

certainly, unless they live alone, we could teach members of their family how to perceive initial and prevent further insulin reactions.

Development of a reaction

The symptoms of hypoglycemia reflect glucose deprivation within the brain. Although physiologists once believed that the brain was limited to glucose as a fuel source, we know now that in starvation the brain is able to utilize ketone bodies for energy. Glucose remains its fundamental fuel, all the same. Although many other body tissues store it, the brain has no stored supply of glycogen. So, a continuous supply of glucose has to cross the blood-brain barrier. Any interference in cerebral circulation, say atherosclerosis, worsens symptoms.

Classically, these symptoms unfold progressively as the various brain structures become involved. They occur in reverse order of phylogenesis: the ''new'' portions of the brain — the cerebral hemispheres and parts of the cerebellum — are the first to suffer from glucose deprivation. These metabolize glucose at the fastest rates.

Lower centers become involved sequentially. The brain structure with the lowest metabolic rate — the medulla oblongata — continues to function long after higher centers have failed. If at last the medulla becomes affected, the patient becomes comatose and obtunded. His breathing and heart rates slow, his temperature drops, his tissue reflexes become

How hypoglycemia affects the brain
The later an area of the brain develops phylogenetically, the greater is its oxygen consumption and need for glucose — and the sooner it is affected by hypoglycemia. Thus the sequence of response is as follows: (1) as the forebrain is affected the patient experiences somnolence, perspiration, hypotonia, and tremor; (2) the thalamus and hypothalamus produce a loss of consciousness; primitive movements, such as sucking, grasping, and grimacing; twitches, restlessness, clonic spasms; hyperresponsiveness to pain; tachycardia; erythema; perspiration; and mydriasis; (3) the midbrain causes tonic spasms, inconjugate ocular deviation, and Babinski's reflex; and in the final phase (4) the effect on the hindbrain induces extensor and flexor spasms when the head is turned, deep coma, shallow respiration, bradycardia, miosis, no pupillary reaction to light, hypothermia, atonia, hyporeflexia, and no corneal reflex.

Physiologic response to hypoglycemia

Brain
Drowsiness, loss of consciousness, convulsions, headaches, aphasia, paralysis, twitching, dizziness, depression, blurred vision

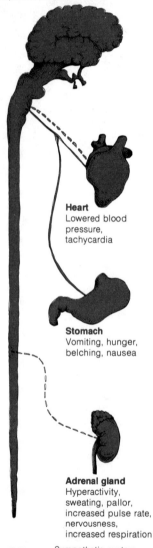

Heart
Lowered blood pressure, tachycardia

Stomach
Vomiting, hunger, belching, nausea

Adrenal gland
Hyperactivity, sweating, pallor, increased pulse rate, nervousness, increased respiration

 ▭▭▭▭ *Sympathetic system*

 ◠◡◠◡ *Parasympathetic system*

depressed, and his pupils contract and become unresponsive. All reflect medullary involvement.

Some researchers attribute the pace of involvement to varying metabolic needs of the different brain parts. Others now believe the forebrain's more complex neurophysiologic connections become depressed by the metabolic insult of glucose deprivation, while the simpler brain stem connections — driven by strong afferent impulses and local chemical stimuli — persist. Either way, the effects of glucose deprivation are marked.

Recognizing a reaction
The physiologic response to lowering the blood glucose level follows this pattern:
- The parasympathetic nervous system becomes excited. *Look for hunger, nausea, eructation, and possibly slowed pulse and lowered blood pressure.*
- Cerebral function declines. *Look for lethargy, lassitude, and yawning.* Conversation may become more of an effort. So may simple calculations.
- In response to need, the sympathetic nervous system releases epinephrine from the adrenal medulla. This stimulates the breakdown of stored liver glycogen into glucose. *Look for sweating, tremor, and cardiac palpitation. Also, look for an increase in blood pressure, heart rate, and respirations.*

During hypoglycemia, this adrenergic response is a valuable one. The liver stores about 75 g of glycogen to be mobilized; epinephrine is a powerful stimulator of liver glycogenolysis, creating an immediate rise in blood glucose concentration. Epinephrine also arouses the reticular-activating system, so the patient is alert and wakeful. But if liver glycogen becomes exhausted without replenishment of glucose from some source, convulsions and coma will follow.

Yet patients taking long-acting and intermediate insulins may not show these classic symptoms of insulin reaction. With these insulins, the slow decline in blood glucose makes cerebral symptoms more pronounced. There may be change in personality, work performance, or study habits. There may even be aphasia, uncoordinated movements, mental deterioration, or psychotic behavior. The symptoms most nearly resemble alcoholic intoxication and sometimes are mistakenly diagnosed as such.

Another hazard: These insulins often reach their peak of action while the patient is asleep. In the diabetic patient under stress, look for nightmares, crying out during sleep, sleepwalking, night sweats, and unusual sleeping postures — all warning signals.

Any misinterpretation delays giving food. And either food by mouth or glucose by injection is the only thing that can ultimately reverse the hypoglycemia and avoid permanent damage.

Assessing a reaction

When the diabetic patient under your care has an insulin reaction, you must assess it thoroughly to try to find its precise cause and also to help the doctor as he determines whether to lower the dose. You will need to know the patient's health history.

Here are several things that can complicate the diabetic patient's normal insulin-glucose metabolism.

Kidney failure: Ordinarily the kidney degrades and excretes about 7 units of insulin every day. But if the kidneys are severely diseased, less than 0.5 unit of insulin may be excreted. This gives the remaining insulin a longer half-life and in effect raises the dose. Keep this in mind, even when kidney disease has not been established, because diabetic patients are prone to renal pathology.

Liver disease: Diabetes doesn't produce any specific liver disease. But acute viral hepatitis and cirrhosis of the liver are often associated with it. Then, the deficiency of hepatic glycogen makes the insulin-dependent diabetic patient more sensitive to his insulin dose.

Alcoholism: Everyone knows that some diabetic patients are also chronic alcoholics. But the combination of injected insulin and excessive alcohol is disastrous. Alcohol prevents gluconeogenesis within the liver; glucose release is inhibited; hypoglycemic coma and irreparable brain damage can result. Since beer and wine contain carbohydrates, the risk with these is lessened.

Medication: Some medications — aspirin in high doses, for example — contribute to insulin hypoglycemia. Find out what drugs the patient is taking and learn which ones have hyperglycemic or hypoglycemic potency.

Aspirin or other salicylates will increase peripheral utilization of glucose and therefore decrease blood glucose. The insulin dose may need to be lowered in an arthritic patient with diabetes taking large doses of aspirin.

Propranolol (Inderal) is another drug with hypoglycemic potential. This beta adrenergic–blocking agent is used for cardiac conditions. But when the diabetic patient taking this drug has an insulin reaction, epinephrine cannot act to increase the glucose output from the liver. The stage is set for a reaction without adrenergic defense to buffer it.

Other drugs can produce a hypoglycemic effect, too, by enhancing hypoglycemic reactions or by producing an intrinsic action. These include certain anabolic steroids; guanethidine (Ismelin); monoamine oxidase (MAO) inhibitors, such as tranylcypromine (Parnate); and certain sulfonamides.

Increased insulin: You should be well acquainted with the Somogyi effect in managing difficulties in diabetes. It works like this: To control rising blood glucose levels, the insulin dose is ordinarily increased. This drops the glucose level, but that in turn calls out epinephrine, adrenal corticosteroids, and growth hormone, all in the body's attempt to oppose the excessive action of the insulin. Epinephrine spurs glycogenolysis in the liver; the corticosteroids stimulate gluconeogenesis. These extra efforts produce rebound hyperglycemia. Watch for nightmares and night sweats and, in the morning, increased urine glucose with ketones present or increased blood glucose on fingerstick. A doctor, mistaking these signs and symptoms for a worsening of the basic diabetes, may inject more insulin and actually aggravate the Somogyi cycle. The appropriate therapy at this stage is to *lower* the insulin dose and return the diabetes to a stabilized state.

When it seems necessary to augment the insulin dose for a diabetic patient who has been following a satisfactory pattern of control up to this point, be sure that the patient and you — the nurse — coordinate your efforts with those of the doctor. Get the patient to record unusual circumstances of symptoms and the times of their occurrence. Reviewing written clues combined with a verbal account makes more sense in patient treatment.

A critical misconception
Bill P., a 22-year-old medical student with diabetes, was hospitalized with a kidney infection and had an initial blood glu-

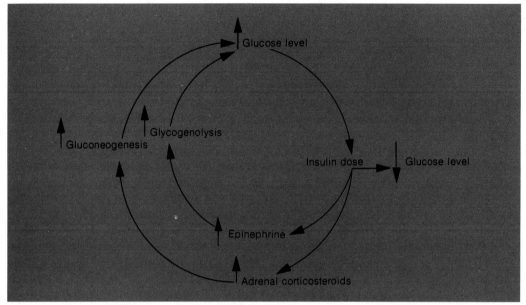

cose reading of 400 mg/dl. Additional insulin had brought it down to 200 mg/dl, almost twice the norm of 60 to 120 mg/dl. Yet the patient was perspiring, trembling, breathing rapidly, and asking for juice to relieve his symptoms. The astute nurse responded to his request, and the symptoms subsided.

Clinical signs don't necessarily correlate with the blood glucose level. Symptoms of hypoglycemia do not depend on an absolute blood glucose reading: they are precipitated by any sudden drop — even from 400 to 200 mg/dl.

To get a quick index of blood glucose level: Put a drop of capillary blood from the patient's fingertip, the earlobe, or a heel puncture on a reagent strip, such as Chemstrip bG. Then after following the instructions given with the product, compare color reaction on the strip with that on a reference color chart. In any case, this method allows for estimations of blood glucose between 40 and 800 mg/dl. But a reflectance photometer, such as the Glucometer, reads the test block electronically and displays a more precise reading.

Remember, the diabetic patient whose circulating glucose has dropped sharply will need food or I.V. glucose to avoid the degenerative effects of insulin reaction.

Prevention: How can nurses help?
Be alert for symptoms. Be mindful of how many varieties of response to hypoglycemia there are and how they vary in the

The Somogyi effect
Some patients who take only one dose of insulin a day have a hypoglycemic reaction by late afternoon only to suffer a rebound hyperglycemia the following morning. Increasing the insulin dosage only aggravates the cycle, as this diagram shows. Splitting the same dosage into several injections during the day eliminates the problem and stabilizes the patient's condition.

Hypoglycemia in review

Hypoglycemia is a dangerous condition. Here's a recap of the primary signs and symptoms.

APPEARANCE:
- Pale
- Staggering gait
- Delirious
- Seizures
- Coma
- Yawning
- Blanching around nose and lips (circumoral pallor)

EYES:
- Crossed
- Dazed
- Dilated pupils

EMOTIONAL RESPONSE:
- Irritable
- Anxious
- Unexpected behavior changes

PHYSICAL RESPONSE:
- Trembly
- Weak
- Drowsy
- Cold, clammy sweat
- Light-headed
- Headache
- Difficulty in talking
- Mouth and tongue numb

CIRCULATION:
- Rapid heart beat
- Strong pulse

URINE SPECIMEN:
- Urine negative for glucose by second voiding

NEUROLOGIC:
- Babinski's reflex often present

individual. Teach your patients the more subtle warnings — lassitude; lethargy; hunger; inability to concentrate, to read, to add figures, to think. These early signals are too often mistaken for being tired. But this is when the patient should eat. Help him recognize this.

Keep regular mealtimes. Diabetic patients and the people closest to them must acknowledge that their actions often set the stage for insulin hypoglycemia. Perhaps you can help them here. To illustrate: Henry P., a 50-year-old businessman, took his 60 units of daily NPH insulin at 8 o'clock one morning. But because he had some abdominal cramping and diarrhea, he didn't eat breakfast. By 10 o'clock he was showing signs of a reaction.

Cheryl M., 19, was trying to crowd too much into a college schedule. She injected her daily morning NPH insulin and ate breakfast. But she didn't finish her lunch because she wanted to get to an exam early. She was unable to complete the exam because her blood glucose level dropped too low.

Situations like these should be thoroughly described to the diabetic patient so he will know to avoid them.

Surprisingly enough, though, hospital routine may be to blame, too. Thomas L., 61, was hospitalized for probable pneumonia and, after his morning insulin, but before breakfast, was hustled off for a diagnostic X-ray. There he waited for 2 hours. He began to feel dull and hungry, and realized he did not have his emergency sugar supply. Just as he was about to go ask for a snack, he was called in for a chest film. He began to shake and perspire. The technician gave him a cup of coffee with sugar. This helped until he returned to his room and breakfast.

Another way we must help the hospitalized patient with diabetes is to bear in mind that his insulin dose may need to be cut as he recovers from a severe illness or from surgery.

Watch out for less food or extra activity. Some patients with diabetes may try to ignore the basic principles of dietary management. First make sure they understand them; then explain the importance of adhering to the diet regimen, which includes eating regularly and on schedule and eating the kinds and amounts of food needed. If the requisite food isn't eaten at a main meal, the remaining ration of carbohydrates, proteins, or fats must be substituted immediately. Snacks are also needed to neutralize insulin absorbed at certain hours.

Whenever exercise or heavy activity is planned, the diabetic patient must either increase his carbohydrate and protein intake or cut down on his insulin. In an adult it may be best to lower the morning insulin that day. A child should increase his food intake.

Avoid dosage errors. The kinds of errors patients can make in dosage or administration of insulin, leading to a reaction, are too numerous to list. Again, by working with the patient, you can help him avoid this.

Be sure the patient knows that most insulin comes in U-100 concentration now. There are patients who, because using the new U-100 insulin means a smaller volume injected than their previous U-40, think that they are not getting enough insulin.

To uncover errors, observe the patient giving himself insulin and checking his own urine for glycosuria or his own blood for glucose at each visit. That's standard practice in many diabetic clinics. I have seen patients misinterpret the urine and blood testing, try to use insulin that has clumped, and mismatch their insulin bottles and boxes. Several times I have found patients reading the unit strength from the box when, in fact, the bottle was of a greater concentration.

Treatment: Reversing the symptoms

The initial treatment for insulin-induced hypoglycemia is 10 g of quick-acting carbohydrate followed by a protein snack. Overloading with carbohydrate actually slows the reversal and "spikes" the blood glucose level.

Many people with diabetes restrict themselves to correction with orange juice. Although 4 oz of orange juice contains the requisite 10 g of carbohydrate and about 6 mEq of potassium, which is also helpful in relieving hypoglycemia, there is no use running around in an emergency to get orange juice when other sweets or sweet drinks are right at hand. The table on page 124 shows several useful foods containing about 10 g of carbohydrate.

The diabetic patient should always carry hard candy, gumdrops, or the equivalent in pocket, purse, or glove compartment. But be sure he understands that, though these foods are right for emergencies, they are not to be freely consumed. Children, in particular, are quick to misuse these emergency foods. Some diabetic patients are better off carrying glucose tablets, marketed as "dextrose tablets" or "dextrose wafers."

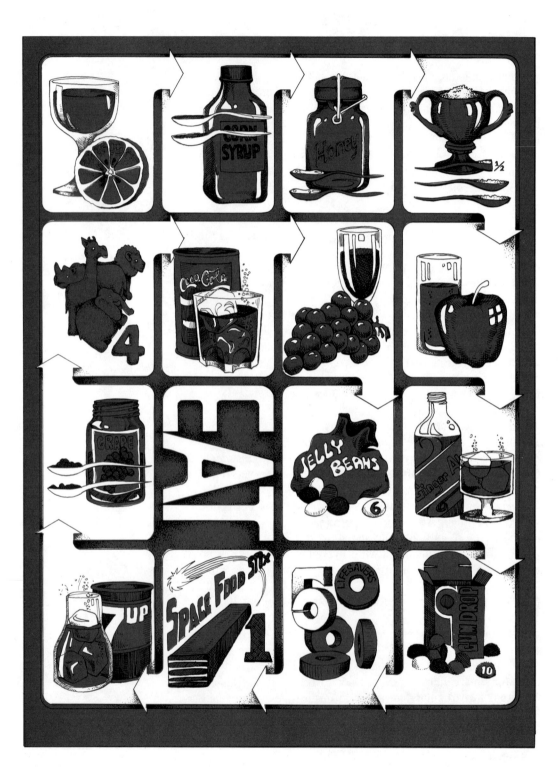

(These are so sweet they're less tempting than candy.) You might also explain that taking fruit juice when they need sugar gives added nutrients not present in the carbonated drinks and candies.

After the patient has responded to the quick-acting carbohydrate, a *supplemental, slowly digestible carbohydrate (for example, milk, cottage cheese, peanut butter, and bread) must be given*. This will maintain the body glucose, restore the liver glycogen, and prevent secondary hypoglycemia.

In severe cases

You can occasionally expect abnormal behavior during an insulin reaction. The person may be agitated. He may spit out food given him. He may spill the juice. But it is unsafe to force food by mouth when his swallowing is impaired: he may aspirate it. Under the circumstances, administering glucagon is the best practice.

This hepatic glycogenolytic substance is produced by the alpha cells of the pancreas. It can be given subcutaneously, intramuscularly, or intravenously. When liver glycogen stores have not been depleted, it will raise the blood glucose level in 5 to 20 minutes. If there is delayed response, one or two additional doses can be given. If there is even minimal glycogen in the liver, it should arouse the person enough for you to give him some food until he is seen by a doctor. Because glucagon's effects last only an hour, and use the liver stores as well, the patient must have extra carbohydrate.

Every patient with diabetes who is taking insulin should have glucagon available in his home and his family should know how to use it. They need to know when to give it, how to mix it, how to give it, and what to do after it has been given. It is a necessity for individuals who develop insulin reactions without warning.

A second emergency tool is epinephrine, 0.5 ml of a 1:1,000 solution (or less than 0.5 ml if it is a small person or a child). This given subcutaneously will stimulate glycogenolysis in the liver, too. But because it also has cardiac effects, it is not safe for everyone.

If the patient hasn't responded to other methods, he needs intravenous glucose. Concentrations of from 10% to 50% are suitable; 50% is most commonly used. The amount required depends on the severity of the hypoglycemia. Response is immediate.

How to treat hypoglycemia
The initial treatment for insulin-induced hypoglycemia is 10 g of quick-acting carbohydrate, such as those shown on the opposite page. Give 4 oz of apple juice, orange juice, or ginger ale; 3 oz of Coca-Cola or 7-Up; or 2 oz of grape juice. Dry measurements are shown in teaspoonfuls.

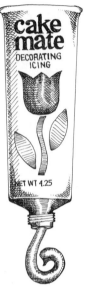

A home remedy
If a patient with hypoglycemia is comatose and you don't have one of the commercial glucose products, you can raise his blood glucose quickly by placing Cake Mate Decorating Icing between his gums and cheeks.

Of course, I.V. injection is usually impossible without trained personnel. For emergency use by the family, there are at least three commercial glucose products prepared in a synthetic base with a gluelike consistency. If the diabetic patient has a reaction and can't swallow, a prescribed amount is squeezed into the mouth. The solution is either absorbed through oral tissues or swallowed by reflex. Then, as the glucose reaches the blood, he may become aroused enough to take some quick-acting carbohydrate food.

These commercial glucose products are *Glutol, Glutose,* and *Instant Glucose.* They come packaged in plastic squeeze bottles or tubes. Because these resemble medicinals, they should be separately stored, though, where they are instantly available. They are convenient because they are easily given. In an emergency where none of these is available, honey could be used on the tongue in small amounts up to 2 teaspoonfuls.

And remember
But we should always avoid the suggestion to someone with diabetes that a medicinal is a remedy for insulin injection. His best treatment is prevention. His best protection is a balance among food intake, exercise, and insulin.

If he has a series of frequent, mild reactions, or a single, moderate reaction — or a severe one — he should check with his doctor before taking the next dose of insulin. This way, both patient and doctor can assess the situation immediately and perhaps adjust the dose.

Remember these important points about insulin reactions:
1. Teach your patient and his family how to recognize early signs of insulin reactions; for example, drowsiness, confusion, and loss of consciousness.
2. Encourage your patient to keep regular mealtimes, to avoid insulin dosage errors, and to be aware that less food or increased exercise may cause hypoglycemic symptoms.
3. Initially treat insulin-induced hypoglycemia by giving 10 g of quick-acting carbohydrate followed by a protein snack.
4. Be aware that a patient experiencing the Somogyi effect will require a lower than usual insulin dose to control his rebound hyperglycemia.

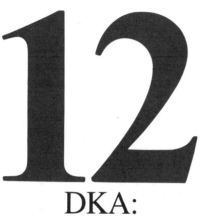

12

DKA:
Breaking a vicious cycle

BY DIANA W. GUTHRIE, RN, PhD, FAAN, AND
RICHARD A. GUTHRIE, MD

OF THE THOUSANDS OF PATIENTS with diabetes mellitus, all but the most stable ones walk a tightrope to avoid two possible upsets — hypoglycemic shock on one hand, ketoacidosis on the other. Diabetic hypoglycemia was covered fully in the last chapter. Now, let's take a good look at its equally acute metabolic opposite, diabetic *ketoacidosis.*

Ketoacidosis arrives by a complex process that may occur in someone newly diabetic, like Donna P. mentioned below, or in someone who has had the disease for a long time. It may come on over a period of weeks, or in a few hours if the diabetes was not previously controlled.

With proper treatment, though, this life-threatening problem should be resolved in 12 to 24 hours. Yet even today, deaths are still reported because the illness is usually so acute, because the patient or his family failed to get help in time, or because a really well-trained medical staff wasn't available.

Patient education, then, is critically important. But so is reliable knowledge of the medical and nursing staff who must deal with this problem. You may find yourself actively involved in both phases. Do you know how to care for such a patient? The following case tells a typical story:

Donna P., a 22-year-old woman previously in good health, was brought to the emergency room one morning by ambulance. She was comatose, with fast, deep, labored breathing. Her breath had the odor of acetone, and she appeared cachexic. More striking was the look of severe dehydration: her eyes seemed sunken, her mouth dry, and her skin loose. Her sister, who accompanied her, confirmed the doctor's suspicion. Although the patient had eaten with increasing appetite over the past few weeks, she had lost an undetermined amount of weight. The sister also confirmed that the patient had shown unusual thirst for several weeks. She reported that Miss P. had seemed increasingly lethargic and depressed lately...had complained of abdominal pains the evening before and vomited once...and had been found barely conscious this morning.

No urine specimen was obtained, but a blood sample was. To save needed time, the blood was tested for glucose in the emergency room with Dextrostix and for acetone with Acetest. The high (greater than 400 mg/dl) glucose reading was later confirmed by the laboratory as 500 mg/dl. The positive serum acetone reading on the Acetest was confirmed by the laboratory.

What was the diagnosis? The polyphagia and polydipsia spelled early uncontrolled diabetes. The cachexia and the dehydration from polyuria represented its progression. The acetone odor and Kussmaul's breathing showed ketoacidosis and the body's attempts to modify it by venting excess carbon dioxide (a chemical breakdown of carbonic acid to carbon dioxide and water) through the lungs. The lethargy, depression, abdominal pain, and vomiting also can go with diabetic ketoacidosis (DKA).

Miss P. was given a bolus dose of 5 units of regular (rapid-acting) insulin and we started an I.V. She was transferred to the intensive care unit — where these critically ill patients belong — for treatment of diabetic ketoacidosis.

How did Donna P., until recently a healthy young woman, get to be so ill? Before we review the treatment given her, it is important to look at the stages of metabolic change that can bring this patient — and others like her — to a critical state.

The road to DKA
Acute insulin deficiency is the cause and the hallmark of DKA. When insulin is lacking in blood and tissue, a vicious cycle begins. The absolute lack of insulin results in high blood

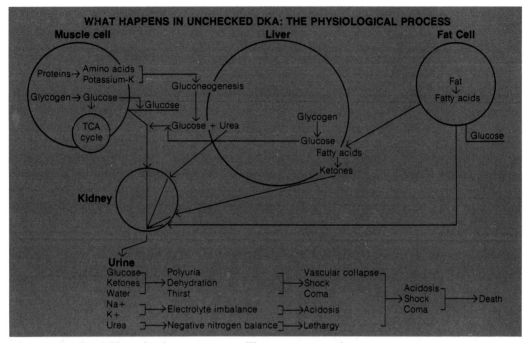

WHAT HAPPENS IN UNCHECKED DKA: THE PHYSIOLOGICAL PROCESS

glucose levels. Although glucose can readily enter nerve tissue, erythrocytes, intestinal mucosa, liver cells, and kidney tubules without it, insulin is essential for the glucose supply of most cells including fat, muscle, fibroblast, mammary glands, the anterior pituitary, the lens of the eye, and the aorta. These cells that need insulin constitute a large percentage of body mass and energy expenditure and perform a large part of the tissue building and repair.

Insulin is also needed to facilitate amino acid anabolism for the protein synthesis of cell building and to stabilize the storage of fat. Without insulin the body enters a serious catabolic state. It happens thus: Glucose, failing to enter the cells, is not converted to energy but accumulates in the blood. When it exceeds the renal threshold, it spills into the urine. The excess blood glucose becomes an osmotic diuretic. So does sodium and potassium loss, taking with them some of the body's bicarbonate stores and preventing the needed formation of further bicarbonate. Bicarbonate is the principal blood base for buffering carbonic acid: when it is used up, acidosis begins.

At the same time, the cells without glucose are beginning to starve and, so, fats are broken down for energy. They are broken down faster than they can be metabolized. That's

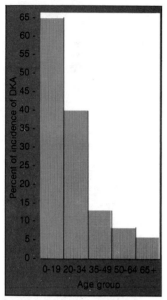

Episodes of DKA and coma
You can see from this graph just how severe and unstable Type I, or insulin-dependent, diabetes is. Many of the young patients suffered episodes of DKA and coma because their conditions went undetected and uncontrolled. Fortunately, the DKA mortality is only 3% to 10%.

because insulin no longer suppresses lipase enzymes, and so, ketone acids, the metabolic products of fat breakdown, accumulate in the circulation.

The body tries to buffer the mounting acidosis. As the renal mechanism for acid excretion (and bicarbonate conservation) is overwhelmed, the respiratory mechanism takes over. The lungs remove carbonic acid by venting carbon dioxide ($H_2CO_3 \rightarrow H_2O + CO_2$). So in metabolic acidosis, the respiratory center is stimulated into the rapid Kussmaul's respiration characteristic of DKA. As long as this mechanism can compensate for acid accumulation, the pH will not decline sharply and the patient may not seem ill. This may happen even though the 20:1 bicarbonate:carbonic acid ratio will actually shift as serum bicarbonate levels decline. But when the lungs' alkalosis can no longer offset the metabolic acidosis, serum pH drops and symptoms develop rapidly.

Protein stores also break down to provide energy to the glucose-deprived cells. But, as with fat, it costs something. The liver, intervening, breaks amino acids into glucose and nitrogen. But without insulin the glucose remains unavailable to the cells and piles up in the blood, intensifying glycosuria, diuresis, and the rest. Nitrogen accumulates, too. Blood urea nitrogen (BUN) levels may rise as urea formation outstrips excretion. And protein breakdown brings marked loss of intracellular potassium, though circulating potassium may be normal or even high.

Many enzyme systems function only within a narrow range of pH. When acidosis depresses their action, the systems — and especially the tricarboxylic acid (TCA) cycle — slow down more and more. Ketones are metabolized increasingly less effectively. Acidosis is enhanced and so is catabolism. The body is now in a state of chronic stress: Impose an acute stress upon it, such as an infection, and the patient quickly deteriorates.

Stress, through its effects of greater adrenocortical steroid output, worsens the existing metabolic alterations. Amino acids cannot be turned into body protein but stimulate the liver to further gluconeogenesis, which breaks the amino acids into more glucose and nitrogen. And the glycerol portion of triglycerides is set free for further gluconeogenesis.

Unless it is interrupted with proper treatment, this cycle of ketosis, acidosis, tissue breakdown, more ketosis, and more acidosis will end in coma and death.

But why the *acute* insulin deficiency? Insulin deficiency, also called Type I diabetes, has no known etiology. However, new data shows that a genetic defect within the body's immune system may be a possible cause. This defect, carried in the HLA (human leukocyte antigen) system on the short arm of the number six chromosome, allows infectious agents (viruses) to damage and subsequently destroy beta cells in the pancreas, resulting in diabetes. As a result, the new and undiagnosed diabetic patient is in a state of chronic insulin deficiency something like that of the poorly controlled known diabetic patient. This is what happened to Donna P.

At this point, one of several things may follow: a state of absolute insulin deficiency may be reached; or, more usually, superimposed stress results in elevated blood glucose levels, which in turn decreases insulin production. The stress may result from emotional trauma, pancreatitis, steroid therapy, Cushing's disease, hemochromatosis, thyroid crisis, or almost any other physical illness; or it may result from infection, surgery, pregnancy, or rapid growth. Or, instead of an insulin deficiency, insulin *resistance* may sharply raise the need for the hormone. Of all these situations, infection and rapid growth are the two most common precipitating causes of DKA. (In the well-insulinized patient, of course, far more stress is required to precipitate acute insulin deficiency than in the one who is chronically insulin-deficient.)

Penalty for stress

Then what was the reason for Donna P.'s sudden acute insulin deficiency? No infection could be found. And the patient, though responding to treatment, was still partly comatose and could not be questioned.

It was her sister who came to the rescue. She recounted that Miss P. had been having a stormy relationship with a man for several months. A few days earlier, after he learned that Miss P. was pregnant with his child, he left for the West Coast with no forwarding address. Donna P., who had obviously been losing a battle with undiagnosed diabetes mellitus for several weeks, possibly because of her pregnancy, was now faced with the emotional upheaval of both pregnancy and desertion. The stress was too much for her, and diabetic ketoacidosis was the result.

Differential diagnosis

How was the staff so sure of the diagnosis? Actually, when all the signs, symptoms, and laboratory values are put together, little else can be confused with DKA. With insulin deficiency, the first result is hyperglycemia. Only a blood glucose test would pick up this symptomless change. Glycosuria follows, and only a urinalysis would reveal it. But then come thirst, polyuria (even up to 3 or 4 gal a day), and inevitable dehydration, after which oliguria may set in. During polyuria, electrolytes are lost in the urine. As sodium and potassium are lost, there will be muscle weakness, extreme fatigue, and malaise. (Potassium depletion can cause cardiac dysrhythmias and arrest. Watch for this problem during treatment as soon as cell repair begins after insulin injection, for treatment may lower the serum potassium too rapidly.)

With fat now breaking down for energy faster than it can be used, ketones (acetoacetic acid, beta-hydroxybutyric acid, and acetone) appear in blood and urine. Acidosis begins, with Kussmaul's respiration following as a compensation. Acetone's fruity odor will be evident on the breath. Often there is abdominal pain simulating acute appendicitis. The cause is unknown, but it may be from electrolyte imbalance and the high fat content of the intestinal tract blood vessels. The patient may vomit, which results in the loss of hydrochloric acid but also sacrifices other electrolytes.

Semistarvation of the cells now brings hunger and increased food intake. Nonetheless, the patient may lose as many as 20 to 30 lb. At last the brain can no longer function under severe dehydration, electrolyte imbalance, and acidosis. The untreated patient becomes comatose.

Look for DKA in any patient who is comatose, obviously dehydrated, and in deep labored respiration. Laboratory values can confirm your suspicions:

• Blood sugar: elevated. Values may range from 350 to more than 2,000 mg/dl, depending upon severity and duration of DKA. Usually between 400 to 800 mg/dl

• Serum ketones: usually elevated to 3 or more dilutions of the serum

• Urine: sugar and acetone both positive

• Serum lipids: elevated, often giving a creamy, opalescent appearance to the serum

• Hematocrit: usually elevated from dehydration

• BUN: usually elevated from tissue destruction and dehydration

• WBC: usually elevated by dehydration, stress, intercurrent infection

• Serum sodium: usually low (despite lowered blood volume)

• Serum potassium: low, normal, or elevated — with *body* potassium markedly decreased.

Despite the distinctiveness of these combined signs and symptoms, very often something else may resemble DKA in the beginning. The following disorders will mimic it most closely:

Renal glycosuria (nondiabetic glycosuria) is free of acetone in the urine. There is no ketosis, and the blood glucose level will be normal or even low.

Salicylate intoxication may fool you for a while: it can give deep, labored respiration and a positive urine test for both glucose *and* acetone. But the blood glucose level is not usually elevated, although the blood and urine salicylate levels are elevated. Because both salicylate and acetone (ketone) give a positive reading on the ketone test, you can make doubly sure by boiling the urine and retesting it; the acetone of DKA will boil away but the salicylate of aspirin poisoning will remain.

Lactic acidosis must be differentiated from DKA, too. Lactic acidosis, though rather rare, can accompany a variety of other metabolic problems, such as salicylate intoxication, ethylene glycol poisoning, methyl alcohol poisoning, paraldehyde poisoning, azotemic renal failure, liver disease — and even ketoacidosis itself as a coexisting disorder. Except in the last, ketonemia will be minimal, but there will be an unmeasured anion, the so-called anion gap, present in the serum in a value *greater* than the normal 12 mEq/liter. Since the extra anions do not represent ketone, they are probably lactate. Most laboratories do not readily measure lactate and pyruvate. But the anion gap can be figured simply by subtracting from the sodium cation concentration the sum of the chloride and bicarbonate anions, the last determined by measuring the serum CO_2 content. With normal values, it would read, 140 mEq/liter serum sodium − (103 mEq/liter serum chloride + 25 mEq/liter CO_2) = 12 mEq/liter unmeasured anions.

When there is underlying disease and you find unexplained

DKA: What to look for
Here's a recap of the signs and symptoms of diabetic ketoacidosis.
Appearance:
• Flushed face
• Weight loss
• Fatigue
• Kussmaul's respiration
• Dry skin
• Coma

Eyes:
• Double or blurred vision
• Soft eyeballs (from dehydration)

Emotional response:
• Irritable

Physical response:
• Fruity smelling breath
• Abdominal cramps
• Nausea and vomiting
• Diarrhea
• Polydipsia
• Polyphagia
• Polyuria
• Headache
• Dyspnea

Circulation:
• Low blood pressure
• Weak and rapid pulse

Urine specimen:
• Urine positive for sugar and acetone

Neurologic
• Normal or absent reflexes

Kussmaul's breathing without hyperglycemia and a consequent sharp drop in serum CO_2 and pH, suspect lactic acidosis. This is treated with large amounts of bicarbonate — *never* its normal precursor, lactate. Watch for this condition in any acidotic patient receiving I.V. therapy, since I.V. fluids often contain lactate.

Hyperglycemic hyperosmolar nonketotic coma (HHNC) is most often present in diabetic patients who have been receiving enough insulin to prevent fat breakdown, but not enough to prevent a mounting hyperglycemia, which may run from 600 mg/dl to above 1,000. The consequent osmotic pressure of the concentrated glucose acts as a diuretic; blood volume is reduced; coma may follow.

This diagnosis can be made in a comatose patient who is markedly hyperglycemic and dehydrated but has little or no ketosis or ketoacidosis. Treatment requires insulin and large amounts of hypotonic fluids, often 10 to 20 liters in the first 24 hours (see Chapter 13 for more details).

Treatment of DKA

Full-blown DKA is an acute medical emergency. What was the treatment given Donna P.? We mentioned she initially received 5 units (0.1 unit/kg) of perfused regular insulin intravenously upon arrival and was transferred to the ICU. In the ED, I.V. fluids of normal saline solution were also begun to correct the dehydration, sodium depletion, and contracted blood volume. Her treatment in the ICU aimed to:
- clear the serum and urine acetone
- reduce the blood glucose (allowing some hyperglycemia)
- correct the dehydration and electrolyte imbalance.

Some hyperglycemia (200 mg/dl) has to be permitted, lest the patient be thrown into hypoglycemic shock — all too easy. In fact, *the patient can pass from hyperglycemia into insulin shock without regaining consciousness.*

The first laboratory tests ordered for Miss P. and their values appear in the chart on the opposite page. Miss P. was also thoroughly examined for some unsuspected causative infection, and a few appropriate cultures were made. But, as we indicated earlier, no infection was found. The Gravindex test for pregnancy was positive.

Even before the laboratory results came, I.V. therapy was started to relieve the obvious dehydration. Normal saline solution

Test Results for Donna P.		
	NORMAL	INITIAL VALUE
Blood glucose	60 to 100 mg/dl	500 mg/dl (350 mg/dl ½ hour post I.V. insulin)
BUN	10 to 20 mg/dl	40 mg/dl
CBC		
Hemoglobin	12 to 16	18
Hematocrit	33% to 45%	50%
WBC	5,000 to 10,000	17,500
Serum ketones	Negative	Elevated to 4 dilutions of serum
pH	7.35 to 7.45	7.28
Serum electrolytes		
Na	136 to 145 mEq/liter	128 mEq/liter
K	3.5 to 5.0 mEq/liter	5 mEq/liter
Cl	100 to 106 mEq/liter	90 mEq/liter
Ca	4.5 to 5.5 mEq/liter	5 mEq/liter
CO_2	22 to 32 mEq/liter	3 mEq/liter
Urinalysis by indwelling catheter:		
Specific gravity	1.015 to 1.025	1.035
pH	5 to 7	4
Reducing sugars	Negative	5% +
Ketone bodies	Negative	Positive

as a plasma expander was used initially. Dextran, blood, or plasma could also have been used, depending on the severity of the vascular collapse. Regular insulin was given again intravenously at the dose of 0.1 unit/kg/hour. Blood glucose was monitored frequently at the bedside by means of Dextrostix with a Glucometer, first every hour; later, as blood glucose values continued to improve, every 2 hours. Results were cross-checked with the laboratory every 4 hours along with electrolyte determination. Although the Dextrostix measurement isn't sharply accurate, it will measure the drops in blood glucose that come with therapy. Also, it's convenient when minutes count.

Every hour the urine was tested for glucose with Clinitest and for acetone with Acetest as a guide to further insulin therapy. At the same time, urine volume was measured as a guide to fluid therapy.

Once renal blood flow and urinary output were established, a multielectrolyte solution containing potassium was given through the I.V. catheter. And a cardiac monitor was used to check on potassium administration. The ICU nurses who

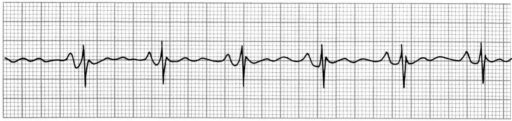

EKG signs of hypokalemia

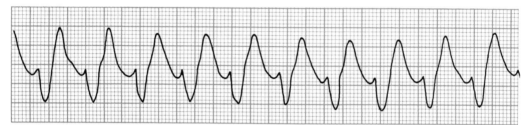

EKG signs of hyperkalemia

looked after Miss P. were trained to recognize the signs of potassium disturbance. (With hyperkalemia, look for tachycardia, then bradycardia; with hypokalemia, dysrhythmia.) Although the I.V. insulin infusion was continued, the administration rate was adjusted to cause a fall in blood glucose levels of 50 to 100 mg/dl/hour.

It may seem surprising, but glucose was added to the I.V. mixture as soon as blood glucose levels fell to 300 mg/dl. This is done because when insulin is supplied, large amounts of circulating glucose are driven into the cells to be normally used again for energy and repair of tissue. But the blood's stores are small compared with the body's needs (plasma is only 5% of body weight). When the blood glucose level comes down to between 400 and 200 mg/dl, depending on how high it has been, 5% or 10% glucose should always be added to the I.V. solution.

The same thing is true of potassium. Once insulin is given, potassium — which has massively shifted out of the cells into the blood and much of that wasted in urine — is then shifted back into the cells again. Moreover, there is a total body deficit of potassium by now even in the hyperkalemic patient. So, with insulin, the serum potassium can drop disastrously. Once the urine is flowing so as to handle the excess, this electrolyte must be given continuously in large amounts. Concentration shouldn't exceed 40 mEq/liter, but on occasion may. The flow rate should be adjusted in relation to the serum potassium values.

No bicarbonate was given to Donna P. In fact, the use of bicarbonate therapy in DKA is controversial. Most authorities have routinely used bicarbonate in large amounts to correct the metabolic acidosis. But others have recently contended that bicarbonate given intravascularly does not cross the blood-brain barrier but merely shifts the bicarbonate:carbonic acid ratio. This releases carbon dioxide, which readily *does* cross the blood-brain barrier and re-dissolves in spinal fluid. That raises the carbonic acid level, enhances cerebral acidosis, and may prolong diabetic coma. Correcting underlying metabolic abnormalities with insulin and I.V. fluids containing electrolytes and glucose is sufficient, unless the acidosis is very severe with a pH less than 7.1 and a serum bicarbonate level less than 7. Then the kidney and lung will correct acidosis in a more physiologic manner. This problem needs further research.

Insulin therapy in DKA

Insulin is the key to DKA therapy. Give as soon as the diagnosis is made. Only regular insulin should be used, never the long-acting forms. The delayed action of Lente and NPH insulins makes them ineffective at the time they are needed and can even make them dangerous later.

One acceptable method of giving insulin to patients with DKA is by low dose I.V. or I.M. administration. In adults, a dose ranging from 3 to 12 units/hour can be safely given by either route. But keep in mind that the best way to calculate insulin dosage — in adults as well as children — is usually by body weight. Give 0.1 unit/kg/hour I.V. as a stat dose and follow it with 0.1 unit/kg/hour I.V. or I.M. Increase or decrease the dose, as needed, to cause a fall of 50 to 100 mg/dl/hour.

DKA treatment: How much insulin and when

When treating DKA, insulin administered I.V. has a more predictable absorption rate than I.M. administration. An insulin infusion pump provides the best assurance that consistent insulin levels are maintained.

When using an infusion pump, administer 2.7 units/hour to a 60-lb child (calculated as 0.1 units/kg/hour) and 2 to 12 units/hour to an adult. Administering insulin on the basis of body

Insulin pumps

Although portable insulin pumps were originally thought to help prevent DKA, some studies show they may increase the risk of this complication. Therefore, portable pump users require frequent blood glucose monitoring.

The pump delivers insulin in small (basal) doses every few minutes and large (bolus) doses on demand. About half the patient's insulin dosage is given in basal doses; the other half in bolus.

The pump can be worn on the patient's belt or kept in his pocket. Most pumps consist of a syringe (to hold the insulin), a syringe plunger, and a mechanism to drive the plunger. When the plunger's depressed, insulin flows from the syringe through the tubing and into the body through a needle inserted subcutaneously.

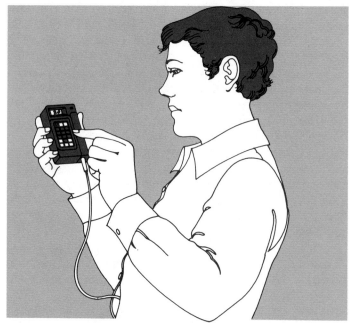

weight is preferable to an absolute dosage.

After the patient's condition has stabilized, give a maintenance dose subcutaneously every 6 hours.

The doses should always be modified upward or downward depending on clinical response and laboratory values of the patient. *No rule or laboratory value can substitute for good clinical judgment.* We find it is always better, too, to underestimate than to overestimate the insulin dose. Smaller, more frequent doses are always safer than larger, less frequent ones. One of the advantages of the I.V. infusion method is that dosages can be changed frequently or discontinued if a rapid rise in blood glucose levels occurs.

Initial fluid treatment for DKA uses such plasma expanders as saline solution, Dextran, plasma albumin, or whole blood. Follow these with "pump priming" solutions of normal saline to expand plasma volume further and establish renal output. Then add potassium and other electrolytes.

Fluid replacements may be calculated in many ways. One of the better ways is to give the patient 2,500 to 3,500 ml of fluid per square meter of body surface area per 24 hours. Use 2,500 ml in the mildly dehydrated patient, and up to 3,500 ml in the severely dehydrated one. These fluids should contain sodium in an amount calculated not only to meet maintenance requirements but to replace deficits. Calculate these by subtracting the actual serum sodium determinants in mEq/liter from 140 mEq/liter of sodium, the normal value, and multiplying by the sodium space, which constitutes about 60% of the body weight in adults and about 70% to 75% in children.

If the patient goes into shock

If the patient passes from hyperglycemia into insulin shock without regaining consciousness, irreparable brain damage may result unless it is recognized and treated promptly. The treatment for insulin shock or hypoglycemia is 50% glucose intravenously.

Once out of acidosis

When Donna P. came out of acidosis, she was given maintenance insulin every 6 hours. Unless a patient's DKA is very mild, the total dose will probably be about ½ to 1 unit/lb (1 to 2 units/kg)/day. Miss P. weighed 110 lb (50 kg) and her insulin dose was 100 units for the first 48 hours postacidosis. This was given in four equal doses during the first 24 hours after her acid-base balance was restored. When a patient is conscious, this should be accompanied ½ hour after each injection by four equal feedings of simple high-carbohydrate nutrients. In Miss P.'s case, the first two feedings were not given because she remained semicomatose and was supported by I.V. therapy.

In fact, with any of these patients, restoring consciousness may take several hours and should not be a major concern. What is of critical importance, though, is for the ICU nurse to recognize the levels of consciousness and recognize symptoms of hypoglycemia. If blood glucose levels are being checked hourly, hypoglycemia should not occur.

After Miss P. did regain full consciousness, her insulin was administered around the meal pattern with three meals and four doses of regular insulin. Her doctors later adjusted this to three doses (regular before breakfast, regular before lunch, and a mixture of regular and NPH before supper) with three meals and a bedtime snack. Before discharge this was changed to two doses per day (16 units of NPH and 8 units of regular insulin ½ hour before breakfast and 6 units of NPH and 6 units of regular insulin ½ hour before supper) with three meals and three between-meal snacks. When using a four-dose insulin schedule, give 35% of the total daily insulin before breakfast, 22% before lunch, 28% before supper, and 15% at midnight. The total daily insulin uptake was adjusted to the previous day's fractional glucose and acetone urine test results and, most importantly, the blood glucose level profile. The so-called *sliding scale* is not rationale therapy because by the time treatment can begin, the blood glucose level is already above acceptable levels. It should never be used. Total daily insulin dosage will gradually decline in the days and weeks after DKA and should be adjusted daily until basal insulin requirements are determined.

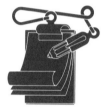

Remember these important points about DKA:
1. Be aware of DKA's cause: Acute insulin deficiency.
2. Look for DKA in any patient who is comatose, obviously dehydrated, and in deep labored respiration.
3. Be careful not to confuse DKA with other conditions that initially resemble it; for example, salicylate intoxication, lactic acidosis, and HHNC.
4. Give regular insulin and fluids as soon as the diagnosis is made.
5. If your patient passes from hyperglycemia into insulin shock without regaining consciousness, administer 50% glucose intravenously to avoid irreparable brain damage.

13

HHNC:
A metabolic hazard

BY KAREN WITT, RN

HAVE YOU HEARD OF HHNC — hyperglycemic hyperosmolar nonketotic coma? It's a widely recognized metabolic derangement, one you may need to recognize to save the lives of certain patients. It can occur as a complication not only of borderline and unrecognized diabetes, but also of a variety of medical and surgical conditions that involve high blood glucose levels and dehydration. Only a few years ago it had a mortality of 60% to 70%. But new treatment protocols have reduced the rate to less than 26%.

Consider the case of Mr. S., who came to our hospital with pancreatic carcinoma. Some months before, Mr. S. had been found to have elevated blood glucose levels. Diet had controlled it until 3 weeks ago, when Mr. S was brought to the hospital with complaints characteristic of pancreatic disease.

Extensive diagnostic studies indicated a pancreatic tumor obstructing the ductal system. Surgeons did a Whipple procedure. They excised the head of the pancreas along with the encircling loop of duodenum. They anastomosed the common bile duct to the remaining duodenum, similarly fastening the stomach to the jejunum — a pancreatoduodenectomy, choledochoduodenostomy, and gastrojejunostomy, respectively. They left an unresectable tumor around his portal vein.

Mr. S. did fairly well after the operation until late evening of the 4th postoperative day. He developed aspiration pneumonia with a fever of 101° F. (38.3 C.), which required Kantrex, Keflin, Solu-Cortef, and supportive respiratory therapy.

By the 5th day his blood gases showed a PaO_2 of 41 mm Hg, well below the normal 80 to 105. Oxygen therapy was started.

Right after the operation, dextrose 5% in water in 0.45% normal saline solution had been given, to which (when urinary flow had returned) potassium chloride was added. These were to keep the fluid and electrolyte balance normal. Also, he had received 10 units of regular insulin daily for 2 days; that was changed to 15 units of NPH insulin daily.

Despite the insulin, and although he did not complain of thirst, Mr. S. was polyuric. His I.V. fluid rate was increased.

By the 6th day, Mr. S. was confused, disoriented, and apprehensive. The nurse discovered him hyperventilating with respirations of 36 breaths/minute. He was lethargic, and he looked dehydrated. She found his blood pressure to be only 96/50 mm Hg; his heart rate, 130 beats/minute. Surely by now the classic picture of diabetic ketoacidosis was emerging. *Yet his serum acetone was still zero.* She notified the doctor.

Lab studies at this point indicated a serum glucose level of 720 mg/dl (far above the normal of 70 to 120) and serum osmolality of 378 mOsm/kg H_2O (above a norm of 275 to 295). With blood glucose levels and serum solutes as high as they were but without acetone, with a pH not acid but indeed a little alkaline — well, what kind of ketoacidosis was this? None at all, as you've surmised. The diagnosis was *hyperglycemic hyperosmolar nonketotic coma.*

On the 6th postoperative day, Mr. S. had received 4,600 ml of I.V. fluid, 1,000 ml of it as normal saline solution during the first 2 hours. On the 7th postoperative day, he received 6,000 ml of I.V. fluids, 1,500 ml of half-normal saline solution with 2.5% fructose and the rest as dextrose 5% in water.

HHNC is a crisis condition: The first concern is to *restore fluid volume and reduce blood glucose.* Mr. S. received 10 units of regular insulin followed by a continuous I.V. insulin drip delivering 6 units/hour until his blood glucose level began to come down. Then he received less frequent doses as he needed them. A Swan-Ganz catheter was inserted to monitor fluid status.

Under more ordinary circumstances, fluid replacement would have been given at a rate no faster than 30 to 40 ml/kg to avoid water intoxication — no more than 3,200 ml/day for

Mr. S.'s Laboratory Values

	NORMAL	ADMISSION	DAY 5	DAY 6	DAY 7	DAY 8	DAY 9	DAY 10	DAY 11
Hematocrit	40-50	42	36			26		40	35
Glucose mg/dl	70-120	274	370	720	459	549	460	525	198
Serum acetone	0	0	0	0	0	0	0	0	0
Urine acetone	0	0	0	0	0	0	0	0	0
BUN mg/dl	6-21	18		49		59	52	52	49
Sodium mEq/liter	134-144		145	164	164	155	151	146	148
Potassium mEq/liter	3.5-5.6		4.3	3.7	4.0	3.4	2.0	2.1	3.1
Chloride mEq/liter	95-105		112	122	130	121	119	109	108
Total bilirubin mg/dl	0.2-0.9	8.6	19.8	14.1	9.7				
Serum osmolality mOsm/kg H_2O	275-295			378	379				
Urine osmolality mOsm/kg H_2O	767-1628			755	810				
Serum albumin g/dl	3.6-5.7	3.6				1.2			
Total protein g/dl	6.6-8.2	6.9	0.5	5.1	5.1	4.4	4.6		5.1
PaO_2 mm Hg	8-105		41	75	58			57	57.4
$PaCO_2$ mm Hg	34-46		24.5	22.5	23.9			49.2	44.1
pH	7.35-7.45		7.58	7.53	7.49			7.38	7.38
HCO_3^- mEq/liter	22-26		22.2	18.4	17.6			28.1	21.5

a man whose preoperative weight was 80 kg (176 lb). But the extreme hyperosmolality and dehydration in HHNC call for extreme measures. So, Mr. S. got a full 10.6 liters in 2 days.

Subcutaneous regular insulin was being continued according to Mr. S.'s blood glucose levels. Insulin added to I.V. solutions is the most rapid form of delivery. But because I.V. solutions can partially inactivate insulin, a slightly higher dose than would be given subcutaneously may be necessary. Oftentimes, I.V. insulin administration is preferred, especially when poor tissue perfusion — such as with a patient in shock — makes a subcutaneous injection ineffective.

Mr. S.'s laboratory values throughout are shown in the table above. On the 8th postoperative day, his plasma proteins dropped markedly (from 5.1 to 4.4 g/dl), so we began giving I.V. albumin. His blood proteins began to climb back toward normal.

A low hematocrit is unusual in patients with HHNC. Mr. S. received 2 units of whole blood because he had a hematocrit of 26, caused by loss of blood from his cancer. After the 8th postoperative day, his blood glucose levels generally came down a little, too. Mr. S. even appeared to be responding despite his hyperosmolar coma. He was more alert and no longer dehydrated.

HHNC: What is it?

The medical and surgical conditions that precipitate HHNC include those that bring on its forerunner, hyperglycemia: diabetes mellitus, pancreatic disease, pancreatectomy, extensive burns, and glucocorticoid therapy, as well as a variety of acute stress conditions. Like corticoid therapy, the latter lead to hyperglycemia through an overproduction of steroids.

Hyperalimentation therapy has sometimes been a factor in HHNC, and so have hemodialysis and peritoneal dialysis, especially when the dialyzing fluid in the latter has a high glucose content or remains in the peritoneal cavity too long. HHNC occurs most often in adults, but occasionally it occurs in children, usually from diabetes, sometimes from heat stroke.

To understand just what happens in HHNC, consider the principles of osmolality, or osmotic pressure, that it involves. In osmosis, fluid naturally crosses a membrane to pass from a weaker solution into a more concentrated one. (Fresh water is always drawn into brine.) Various fluid compartments of the body continually establish osmotic equilibrium in this way.

Normally, sodium exerts most of the osmotic pressure in the body's extracellular fluid, and potassium in the intracellular fluid. Still, those solutes that least quickly penetrate cell membranes have the greatest osmotic pressure, meaning that they most readily draw fluid to themselves, and one of these is glucose. Its molecule is simply too big to get through a cell wall easily. As a result, by remaining where it is, it can attract large shifts of water.

In the pronounced hyperglycemia of HHNC, some of the isotonic intracellular fluid (ICF) is inevitably drawn out to help equalize the growing osmotic pressure of blood now hypertonic with glucose. Water in the ICF moves out of the cell walls into the bloodstream, after a while leaving the cells themselves shrunken and dehydrated.

Osmosis compromised. But without sufficient water from the outside as well, the HHNC patient's blood becomes yet more concentrated, and its volume further depleted. Because, without extra insulin as needed to lower blood glucose levels, osmotic diuresis takes place.

How? In normal osmolar mechanics, large amounts of body water are reabsorbed from the kidney's distal tubules and collecting ducts. This water, drawn out of the urine that is constantly being formed in the tubules, is restored to the blood:

It is extracted by sodium concentrated in the interstitial tissue surrounding the tubules.

But in HHNC, when the plasma osmolality is practically as high as that of these water-absorbing tissues, osmosis cannot draw back the water from the kidney into the blood: There is not a steep enough osmotic gradient. The water is excreted. And the antidiuretic hormone, though called forth by both hyperosmolality and depleted blood volume, can no longer prevent its loss through tubules whose very means of operating — osmotic pressure — have been cancelled out.

But then something else happens. With this wasting of water, the ensuing hypovolemia decreases renal blood flow. This conserves urine, preserving the remaining extracellular fluid volume. That this oliguria reduces water loss is helpful, but it also severely hampers the kidney's excretion of glucose. Without treatment by insulin and fluids, the process becomes self-perpetuating.

The role of glucocorticoids. Several of the conditions preceding HHNC are often treated with glucocorticoids. But glucocorticoids may even initiate the hyperglycemia (and consequently the water diuresis and so the dehydration) through fostering gluconeogenesis and depressing carbohydrate oxidation, as they are known to do. "Steroid diabetes" may in fact persist for some time after steroids are withdrawn. Glucocorticoids may also inhibit the release of the antidiuretic hormone. And possibly they reduce the capacity of the tubule to reabsorb water and solutes, promoting diuresis yet a third way.

The onset of HHNC is typically insidious, as it was for Mr. S. Once HHNC develops, it moves rapidly to a crisis. Early signs in an alert patient usually include polyuria, increased thirst, and a growing impairment of consciousness. Of course, as you are probably thinking, these signs are commonly observed in seriously ill patients of all sorts. And then very often you don't have even these signs to go by because the patients are obtunded or even comatose. But this is why it's medically important to monitor susceptible patients closely with frequent determinations of blood glucose and electrolyte levels.

Failure to recognize the *risk* of HHNC, or to know the syndrome itself when it does come, is bound to contribute to its high mortality. But the one big thing about this disor-

Harbingers of HHNC

Usually HHNC occurs spontaneously. But it may be precipitated by the following:
- cortisol-type steroids
- phenytoin
- antimetabolites
- diazoxide
- propranolol
- high carbohydrate intake in burns
- diuretics, such as thiazides, chlorthalidone, and furosemide.

HHNC can also develop in association with spontaneous Cushing's syndrome and other endocrinopathies.

Terminology

Hyperglycemia — more glucose in the blood than normal.

Hyperosmolality — abnormal concentration; hyperosmolar blood contains more glucose, electrolytes, or other solutes than normal.

Hypovolemia — reduced blood volume; if the patient has not lost blood, he has lost water or shifted it into the cells; the blood is consequently also apt to be hyperosmolar.

Osmolality — strength or osmotic effectiveness, written as milliosmols/kilogram of solvent (mOsm/kg).

Osmosis — a natural principle in which a solvent (for example, water) passes through a membrane from a dilute solution into a more concentrated one.

Osmotic diuresis — excessive water loss through the kidneys; an excess of solutes in the renal tubules forces water excretion so as to carry them off.

Osmotic gradient — the contrast between the osmolality of one solution and another.

Osmotic pressure — the ability of a solution to draw water from another solution across a cell wall, eventually equalizing the concentration of both.

Tonicity — osmotic pressure once again, usually expressed as a physiologic norm: A hypotonic solution contains fewer solutes than blood; an isotonic solution contains them equally; and a hypertonic solution is more concentrated than blood.

der that sets it apart from diabetic ketoacidosis (DKA) and other hyperglycemia-related conditions is either *minimal ketoacidosis or none at all.*

If we look more closely at the separate features of the syndrome, we can begin to put it together better.

Hyperglycemia

The most dramatic finding in HHNC is hyperglycemia, linked with the hyperosmolality responsible for coma. Fasting blood glucose levels may range from 600 mg/dl to 3,000 mg/dl! This high range is usually reached either because of some breakdown in glucose metabolism or more glucose being supplied to the body than the body can burn.

Clearly there is faulty glucose metabolism in diabetes mellitus and in certain cases of pancreatic dysfunction. In patients with acute pancreatic disease, the curtailed supply of endogenous insulin helps elevate the glucose level. In those with known diabetes, and in those who have undergone a pancreatectomy, receiving too little insulin can be the cause.

In patients with severe infection or some other acute stress, or in those receiving glucocorticoids, you will find the blood glucose rising through gluconeogenesis. This synthesis of glucose from protein or fat is a natural effect of the adrenal cortex hormones.

In addition, steroids increase the body's resistance to the action of insulin. With this double-barreled effect in mind, you must be extremely vigilant when glucocorticoids are used with a patient such as Mr. S., or with any patient who may be predisposed to HHNC.

In burn cases, in hemodialysis, in peritoneal dialysis (when high glucose concentrations are used as the dialyzing fluid and remain long enough for the large glucose molecules to be absorbed), as well as in hyperalimentation therapy, patients may receive more glucose than they can metabolize. In hyperalimentation, the prolonged infusion of high glucose concentrations can lead to pancreatic fatigue because of the sharp, continuous demand on the beta cells to produce insulin. If there is at last too little insulin for all the glucose to be used in the tissues, it accumulates in the blood. When the buildup is sufficiently prolonged, the hyperglycemia will lead to actual degenerative changes in the beta cells. Meanwhile, the HHNC syndrome can develop all too quickly if too little supplemental water is given the patient to permit excretion of the glucose by the kidneys: he becomes dehydrated. Be especially wary of dehydration in a patient who cannot complain of thirst.

The blood glucose level is usually lowered with regular insulin. Because patients with HHNC are not generally as insulin-resistant as DKA patients, and because there may be severe body fluid derangements, small and probably frequent doses are recommended. But there is one more thing to watch for in these patients whose metabolism has gotten out of hand: Their blood glucose level is quite labile. You must monitor them closely, watching a narrow line between soaring glucose levels and insulin shock.

Dehydration and hyperosmolality

No one seems sure whether the dehydration leads to hyperosmolality — high concentration of solutes in the blood — or whether the hyperosmolality dehydrates by causing an osmotic diuresis, as it unmistakably does. No matter which, consider volume depletion and hyperosmolality together as the most serious part of HHNC because they can lead directly to hypovolemic shock.

Under this threat, then, the correction of each one — relieving the dehydration and diluting the hypertonicity of the blood — is crucial. Logically, it would seem that hypotonic solutions ought to do the job fastest and best: indeed some authorities have recommended this. Yet it's safe to assume that through osmotic diuresis the patient has lost large total quantities not only of water, but of sodium, potassium, and accompanying anions — despite the probably high serum concentrations of those that remain. Consequently, the use of isotonic saline solution can help repair these absolute deficits. But, more important, it can do something else: *It can help prevent a shift of water back into the intracellular fluid,* whose relatively high concentration might otherwise withdraw the incoming water from the blood and perpetuate hyperosmolality.

On this basis, here's a three-stage plan for therapy:

• *Correct the sodium deficit.* First, correct the sodium deficit as rapidly as possible without overshooting the mark; many of these patients are elderly, remember, and may have heart disease. For Mr. S., you will recall, this correction consisted of 1 liter of normal saline solution over the first 2 hours.

• *Correct the water deficit.* Second, correct the water

Hydrate at the right rate

Your first and most important step in treating HHNC is to hydrate the patient as quickly as possible. Initially, you should use normal saline solution to reexpand volume. Later, you may use a combination of normal saline solution and dextrose 5% in water solution (see top chart at right for secondary hydrating solutions). But remember that a low NaCl concentration must be used with cardiac patients. Use the bottom chart to calculate the rate of flow.

Secondary hydrating solutions		
	mEq/Liter	
DESCRIPTION	Na	Cl
Dextrose 5% in water and 0.33% sodium chloride injection	56	56
Dextrose 2.5% in water and 0.45% sodium chloride injection	77	77
Dextrose 5% in water and 0.45% sodium chloride injection	77	77
Dextrose 5% in water and 0.2% sodium chloride injection	34	34

Dosage and rate of administration (based on 10 drops/ml)				
WEIGHT		APPROX. DOSE	RATE	
lb	kg	ml	ml/min	drop/min
6.6	3	75	1.6	16
8.8	4	90	2.0	20
11.0	5	105	2.3	23
13.2	6	120	2.5	25
15.4	7	135	3.0	30
17.6	8	150	3.5	35
19.8	9	160	3.5	35
22.0	10	175	4.0	40
24.2	11	185	4.0	40
26.4	12	200	4.5	45
33.0	15	230	5.0	50
44.0	20	300	6.5	65
55.0	25	340	7.5	75
66.0	30	375	8.5	85
77.0	35	425	9.5	95
88.0	40	450	10.0	100
99.0	45	500	11.0	110
110.0	50	550	12.0	120
121.0	55	575	13.0	130
132.0	60	600	13.5	135
143.0	65	650	14.0	140
154.0	70	675	15.0	150
165.0	75	700	16.0	160
176.0	80	725	16.0	160
187.0	85	750	16.5	165
198.0	90	775	17.0	170
209.0	95	775	17.0	170
220.0	100	800	17.5	175
231.0	105	825	18.0	180

deficit rapidly, although incompletely. For this, hypotonic fluid is used, rehydrating the patient and yet reducing hyperosmolality faster than added isotonic solution would. The amount of hypotonic fluid needed by an individual to replace water deficit is based upon a comparison of effective and actual plasma osmolality.

In giving hypotonic solution, you must monitor the serum osmolality to prevent that shift of water back into the cells. Although 0.45% saline solution alone is often used for the hypotonic I.V. infusion, some doctors prefer 2.5% fructose in 0.45% saline solution until the blood glucose level drops considerably. Fructose is rapidly absorbed from the blood, chiefly by the liver, and so does not contribute either to plasma tonicity or to osmotic diuresis. During the second stage of fluid therapy, Mr. S. received 0.45% saline solution with 2.5% fructose and dextrose 5% in water.

• *Cautiously return to normal levels of fluid and electrolytes.* On the 9th postoperative day, Mr S.'s potassium losses were great enough (serum potassium was down to 2.0 mEq/liter; see chart on page 143). To require adding 60 mEq of KCl/liter to the I.V., or 120 mEq/day. Of course, the serum electrolyte values don't always tell the true state of bodily derangement. For example, serum potassium levels can be high when the blood has borrowed potassium heavily from the cells, where nearly all of it is stored and used. But the kidneys cannot conserve potassium well. So as soon as the blood's borrowed stores have been partly excreted, the patient will become hypokalemic. By this time, the body may be critically short of its principal electrolyte. Serum potassium levels can also be high in this syndrome when the patient is going into shock, so you should follow these serum values closely in managing the patient. But remember, they're only indicators, not absolutes.

The potassium shift is facilitated by glucocorticoids, either secreted or given. Not only the stress of Mr. S.'s condition, for example, but also the Solu-Cortef that he received must have helped send potassium from cell to serum in the body's effort to keep the latter's levels normal — though they were then lowered by the continuing diuresis of hyperglycemia. Sodium is wasted by the diuresis, too. But proportionately more water is lost, so that Mr. S.'s hypernatremia was primarily a reflection of his dehydration.

Elevated blood urea nitrogen (BUN) is a common finding

in patients with HHNC. Mr. S.'s BUN level rose after surgery from a normal 18 to above 59 mg/dl. This increase in serum urea nitrogen comes not only from dehydration but often, where there is stress or when glucocorticoids are given, from increased protein catabolism. And incidentally, protein breakdown intensifies the loss of cellular potassium.

Nonketosis

Only the absence of ketoacidosis differentiates HHNC from a regular diabetic coma. When all the signs of DKA are there but this one — particularly when the glucose is elevated — that should alert you immediately to the true diagnosis.

What happens in DKA is this: The strongly acidic ketones, including acetone, are formed in the liver out of mobilized fat. Normally, after suitable enzyme changes, they are oxidized only for supplemental energy by the tissues, and unless insulin is lacking, they are formed no faster than they can be used. But without insulin (and so with glucose unavailable as energy to the cells), they are called out in force and pile up in the blood as acetoacetic acid, a derivative, faster than coenzyme A can process it.

What happens in HHNC, according to one theory, is this: The patient has enough insulin to avoid ketosis because the portal vein carries a critical amount from the pancreas to the liver, but still too little to reduce the hyperglycemia that is the earmark of this disease. The hyperglycemia, which induces diuresis, produces hyperosmolar blood, but there is no excessive production of ketone bodies and, therefore, no ketoacidosis.

It's also possible that both glucocorticoids and dehydration have an antiketogenic effect. Glucocorticoids, when given or when produced by the body under stress, promote the synthesis of glucose from fats or from proteins. But the glucose without insulin does not nourish the cells; it merely raises the blood glucose level, intensifies the diuresis, and heightens the hyperosmolality. The vicious circle closes.

Coma

Coma comes insidiously in HHNC. It seems to be the result of both the dehydration and the hyperosmolarity. Cerebral symptoms are probably due to fluid space and electrolyte derangements. Seizures have been reported during the acute phase of HHNC.

Presence of ketone bodies	**Insulin levels**	**Serum growth hormone and cortical levels**
HHNC Minimal ketosis: acidosis, when present, develops from uremia  DKA Sufficient ketone bodies to produce metabolic acidosis (In both types of coma, keep in mind the possibility of lactic acidosis as a complication.)	HHNC Some residual ability to secrete insulin DKA Zero	HHNC Low (may be normal, but lipid-mobilizing effects are minimal or absent) DKA High

Central nervous system manifestation	**Mortality**
HHNC Frequent manifestations other than stupor and coma, including repetitive focal motor seizures, CVA, and other neurologic dysfunction DKA Less frequent manifestations other than stupor and coma	HHNC About 50% because of older age of patients and complications (pneumonia, pancreatitis, thrombosis, cerebrovascular lesions, etc.) DKA As low as zero

Nursing care: Hydration and sensorium

Here are ways you can help prevent HHNC, and ways to help treat it effectively if it does occur.

• *Know your patient.* Know the pathophysiology of his medical problem. Know which patients are going to run a high *risk* of metabolic coma.

• *Maintain hydration.* To prevent dehydration, record intake and output scrupulously. Record daily weight, preferably on an in-bed scale. Notice the degree of skin turgor and mucosal moistness: loose skin and dry mouth are both signs of dehydration. Hypotension and tachycardia are *later* signs of dehydration.

You face particular problems with patients who can't complain of thirst, with elderly ones whose sense of thirst is dulled, and with those who are being hyperalimented or tube-fed. Make sure that they get enough water. Usually, it's up to you to assess change and detect need in any of these susceptible patients.

• *Keep a close check on sensorium.* Changes may be subtle. That's why we advise having the same nursing staff regularly

How HHNC compares with DKA
Although initially the symptoms of HHNC seem similar to those of DKA, understanding the basic differences will help you help your patient.

care for the patient — so they can detect change more easily. Lethargy or confusion indicates a hyperosmolar state.

If HHNC does develop, the nursing care plan will be essentially the same, but now the emphasis will be on replacement and rehydration. You must understand the doctor's rationale in the plan for fluid administration so you can knowledgeably participate and monitor progress.

During the first phase, when isotonic fluids are given rather rapidly to replace blood volume and sodium deficits, be sure the Swan-Ganz line is functioning properly and the flow rate is accurate. Watch the vital signs. *Stabilization of blood pressure will indicate restored volume.* During this period, measure urine output every hour.

During the second phase, that of rehydration, when the emphasis is on water replacement and the concern is for fluid overload, you have to monitor things very closely. A volumetric pump can give needed control in the rate of fluid administration. Be sure to check serum osmolality regularly and report any sudden or dramatic decrease to the doctor at once. Again, observe the sensorium. Its sudden deterioration might warn of cerebral edema.

Nursing care: Glucose and acetone levels
When you have identified your high-risk patients for HHNC, you can help protect them against it by monitoring blood for glucose and urine for acetone. Blood glucose and urine testing should be done on a regular schedule for consistency of test result interpretation.

Making the difference
High blood glucose and glycosuria but *no* acetone, or only a trace, and *no* acidosis — these are what separate HHNC from DKA. (Lactic acidosis, another acidotic condition that can lead to coma, shows no acetone, either. But like DKA, it produces a low pH reading.)

Treatment differs, too, between HHNC and DKA. In DKA, *insulin* is the key. Smaller amounts of fluid are needed to correct the correspondingly milder hyperosmolality of the blood.

In HHNC, insulin is used sparingly: *water* is the key. Once the lost electrolytes are replaced with normal solutions, the quantities of hypotonic intravenous infusion also needed may bring the total fluids given to *10 or 20 liters during the first 48 hours*. When the hydration problem is solved, insulin may be given more freely.

In fact, giving ample water may easily be the key to preventing this syndrome. All too often, when a patient's metabolic status is fluctuating — not only through imbalances of his own illness, but through the health-care team's continuous efforts to regulate them — something can go awry. What goes awry to play its part in HHNC is *dehydration*.

Keep constantly on the lookout for it among your susceptible patients — usually the elderly, the debilitated, the mild or even unsuspected diabetic patients. These are the ones most apt to die. Look to see that their arms and legs are not flabby with newly loose skin, that their face is not pinched and their tongue not dry. Then, too, you should watch for another constant danger: water intoxication. For as soon as glucose levels are reduced, the hyperosmolality of the blood is sharply reduced. This is when water is apt to be drawn into tissues, especially the brain. *The closest observation is necessary*. Because you are the one constantly on the scene, your observations are most important to the patient. If we are *all* alert to it, a hyperosmolar crisis need not usually develop out of some simple decompensation.

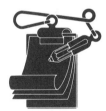

Remember these important points about HHNC:
1. Following diagnosis, restore fluid volume and reduce blood glucose levels.
2. Know that although HHNC occurs most often in adults, it does occur occasionally in children — in most cases, as a result of diabetes, and sometimes from heat stroke.
3. Realize that minimal or no ketoacidosis sets HHNC apart from DKA and other hyperglycemia-related conditions.
4. Treat dehydration and hyperosmolality by correcting the patient's sodium and water deficits and cautiously returning all other fluid and electrolyte levels to normal ranges.
5. Understand that in treating HHNC, insulin is used sparingly: Water is the key.

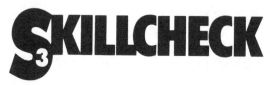

SKILLCHECK

1. Frank Masullo has come to the doctor for a checkup. He mentions that he is concerned because urine test results with reagent strips show 1% to 2% glucose. Yet he insists that he hasn't made any changes in his insulin, diet, or activity. The doctor checks the injection sites on Frank's arms and thighs. Why does the doctor do that?

2. Edwin Allen, a 72-year-old delegate to a convention, has been found staggering up and down the halls of his hotel at 4:30 in the afternoon. When summoned to the scene, the hotel manager gently offers to show Mr. Allen to his room. Mr. Allen becomes hostile and combative, saying that no one is going to lock him up in "this old folks' home." The manager, assuming that Mr. Allen is drunk, calls the police. They, fortunately, discover Mr. Allen's Medic-alert bracelet identifying him as a diabetic and bring him to the emergency department. You find a Medic-alert card in Mr. Allen's wallet stating that he takes NPH insulin and has arteriosclerotic heart disease. What would you deduce about Mr. Allen's condition?

3. Margaret Morris has been hospitalized for diabetic ketoacidosis. Her blood glucose level on admission was 800 mg/dl, her urine contained ketones and 2% glucose, and her electrolytes read Na 125 mEq/liter, K 6.5 mEq/liter, Cl 90 mEq/liter, and CO_2 3 mEq/liter. Her output is way below normal, her face is flushed, and her blood pressure reads 80/58. What would you expect her treatment to be?

4. Andrew Sims appears in the emergency room with the following symptoms: fruity smell on breath, flushed face, profuse sweating, strong but slow pulse, dilated pupils, and confusion about where he is. When you check for identification, you discover from his Medic-alert bracelet that he is diabetic. What would you expect his diagnosis to be?

5. Jamie, age 2, was admitted to the pediatric unit with the following: inflamed throat, fever of 100° to 101° F. (37.8° to 38.3° C.) for 3 days, vomiting and anorexia for 3 days, ex-

cessive urination for 4 days, and polydipsia for 1 day. His blood glucose level on admission was 1,720 mg/dl. His urine contained no ketone. What kind of crisis has Jamie suffered? What fostered it?

6. Anne Loomis, age 25, has just discovered that she has diabetes. When you give her a diet chart, she says she can't read it. She explains that her vision has been blurred recently and that she's afraid she's losing her sight. What would you tell her?

7. Seventy-year-old George Franklin, who has arteriosclerotic heart disease and hypertension, was admitted to the hospital for diagnosis and treatment of extensive skin lesions. The dermatologist prescribed 120 mg of oral prednisone daily. Mr. Franklin also is receiving dextrose 5% in water at the rate of 1 liter every 24 hours. After the 3rd day of treatment, Mr. Franklin becomes disoriented; his blood glucose level rises to 354 mg/dl. You give him 20 units of Lente insulin, as prescribed by the doctor, but 8 hours later Mr. Franklin's blood glucose level has climbed to 1,340 mg/dl. His urine tests are negative for acetone; serum osmolality is 323 mOsm/kg H_2O. Clearly, Mr. Franklin is experiencing HHNC. What do you think precipitated it?

8. Vicki James, your 18-year-old next-door neighbor, was recently hospitalized and diagnosed as diabetic. She was sent home with a diabetic emergency kit containing glucagon, epinephrine 1:1,000 with syringe, dextrose wafers, and Glutose. This afternoon she has appeared at your back door with her kit and says she thinks she's having an insulin reaction. She doesn't know what to use from her kit. What would you advise her?

(Answers begin on page 206)

HOW TO HELP SPECIAL PATIENTS

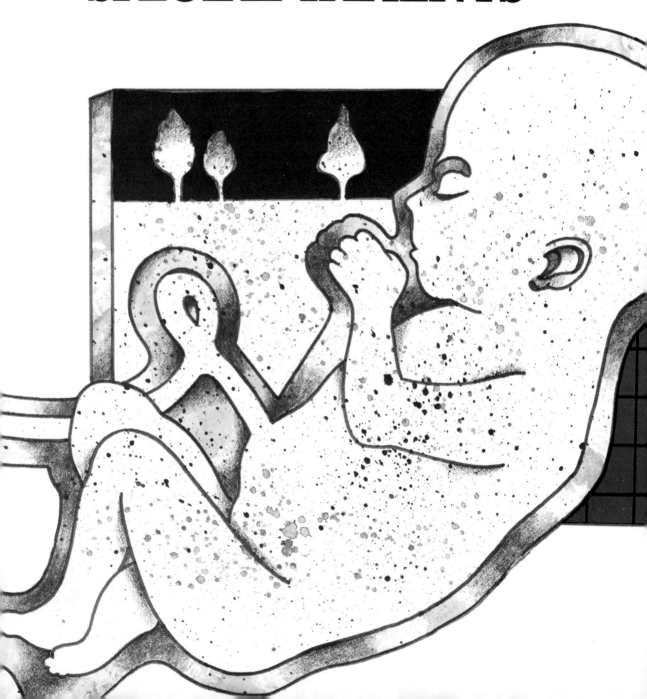

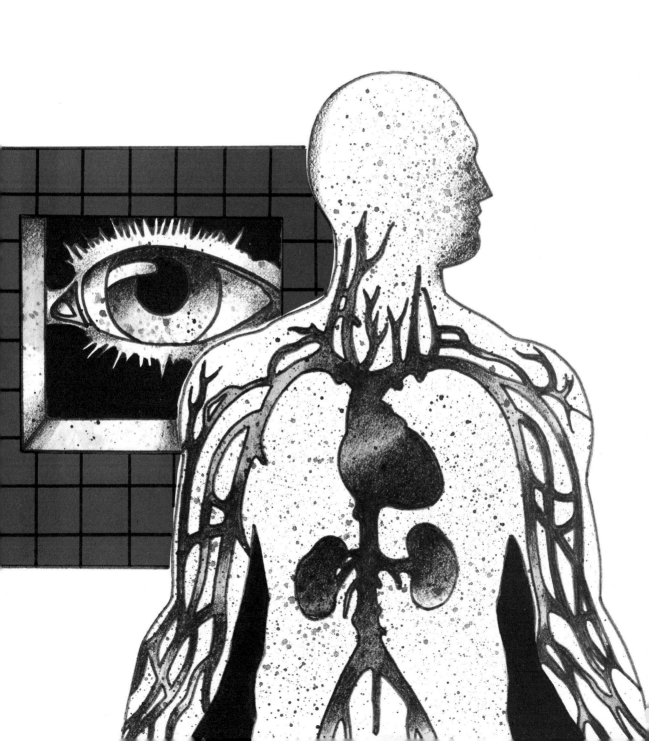

What nursing actions can you take to help
family members overcome their fear of
administering an insulin injection?

What meal and snack patterns usually
work best for a diabetic child?

If your diabetic patient is pregnant,
what are the risks to the baby?

What complications
of pregnancy occur more frequently
in women with diabetes?

What precautions can a blind patient
with diabetes take to guard
against getting a large air bubble
in his insulin syringe?

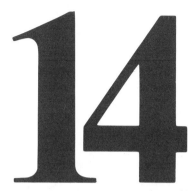

Diabetic children:
Preparing them to live

BY DIANA W. GUTHRIE, RN, PhD, FAAN

NOBODY NEEDS TO TELL you to manage a diabetic child differently than you would a diabetic adult. The child's age alone and his sure dependency on insulin obviously make his needs different.

But the differences run even deeper than that — all the way to minute modifications in diet and insulin dosages to account for the child's size and growth spurts when treating hypoglycemia. In short, you've got to manage the diabetic child realistically: as a typical diabetic patient with some special needs.

Here at the Kansas Regional Diabetes Center, we believe in close metabolic control of diabetic patients. Winegrad, Spiro, and Jackson have shown the need for precise control to avoid later vascular, kidney, and optic-tissue deterioration. Numerous others have shown an inverse correlation between control and early development of vascular disease. No one has proven beyond all doubt that a high level of metabolic control prevents vascular disease or that poor control causes it. But several years ago the American Diabetes Association stated that normalizing blood glucose levels would prevent or delay microvascular disease. With this in mind, we continue to attempt 24-hour control of glycemia and complete "insulinization" of the tissues. We check blood glucose levels four to six times a day and frequently change insulin dosages.

Every child with diabetes should receive *insulin* as soon as the diagnosis is confirmed. Oral hypoglycemic agents should not be used when treating a diabetic child; they eventually only further deplete the pancreas. The child with diabetes probably already secretes little insulin, if any. There is some evidence, however, that giving him insulin early helps restore his own insulin-making ability. The earlier the diagnosis is made, the lower the insulin dose he will need and the easier control will be without hypoglycemia.

The child should be hospitalized during his initial regulation. That enables treating any complications, such as infection or ketoacidosis, and also returning him to a good nutritional status. It also enables determining how much insulin he needs for maintenance and educating both him and his parents in his care. If a young patient is undernourished, he may have to stay hospitalized for some weeks.

The untreated child will have depleted his nutritional stores; in the initial phase of therapy he must build them back. This period of metabolic repletion calls for both more insulin and more food than he will later need for maintenance. Once repletion is over with, his insulin requirements will fall back to those needed for energy and growth. His insulin needs may go down to 0.2 to 0.4 unit/kg of body weight, or about 5 to 10 units a day. If this "honeymoon period" doesn't occur at all, he may stabilize at about 0.6 to 1.0 unit/kg.

We have found that at least two injections a day of a mixture of rapid-acting and intermediate insulin are the best stabilizing doses for children used to eating normal meals and snacks. In fact, for an adolescent boy in the growth spurt, there is probably no other way to keep him satisfied. With a proportionately smaller stomach in which to contain higher caloric needs, the growing child does best, we find, with three meals and three between-meal snacks.

The nature of the disease
Understandably, parents may be upset when they learn that their child has diabetes. However, simply explain to them that from now on another part of the child's life chemistry must be outwardly managed, just like eating, drinking, and excretion. Let them get over the shock of the diagnosis while helping them all you can. Then go over the steps of the young patient's regimen with them, with the patient himself, and with

any interested older brothers and sisters.

Because Type I diabetes is fraught with peril, we cannot teach only syringe care and insulin action. We must spell out what its antagonists are and what situations call them forth. Such antagonists include hormones like glucocorticoids; catecholamines from stress; glucagon as a natural counteragent produced by the pancreas; and growth and thyroid hormones. Trauma, infection, exposure to cold, and running a fever also increase insulin requirement. When the diabetic patient exercises, he must decrease his insulin dosage or increase his food intake.

Diabetes is always difficult to regulate when the patient is upset. The adrenal hormones — the catecholamines — sharply increase the need for insulin. But raising the insulin dosage can invite hypoglycemia because the insulin supply may find itself outstripping its counteragents. Then the body will bend all its chemical efforts to raise the blood glucose level through releasing more counteragents. This can set up an insulin resistance that can only be met with more insulin. Hence — a troublesome trip on the physiologic roller coaster that gives Type I diabetes the name ''brittle.'' Skimping on snacks, increasing exercise, or unwisely increasing insulin can have the same effect if they start the pendulum to swing. Then the child will need a decrease in insulin or redistribution of food intake. Parents should learn to understand when these changes are worth the doctor's attention.

Soon after hospitalization, every child at our hospital receives a diabetic instruction kit containing:

- glucagon
- mixing bottles (if needed)
- insulin (U-100)
- vial of diluting fluid for U-25 or U-50 insulin
- pumice stone, clipper, orange stick, emery boards
- test tube and dropper
- alcohol wipes
- variety of syringes, U-100, or Lo Dose syringes that measure up to 50 units of U-10 insulin, if needed
- pad of paper, pencil
- identification cards and jewelry
- Clinitest and Acetest; equipment for blood glucose self-monitoring
- Clinitest card, 2-drop method, or recording cards and reagent strips.

Testing a sibling for diabetes

Have the mother begin the test when the child's bladder is empty. Give a child over 6 years old 8 oz of orange juice or 4 oz of grape juice, each with 1 tablespoon of sugar added. Follow it in 20 minutes by 6 oz of cola.

Give a child under 6 years old one half the above, except add a full tablespoon of sugar to the fruit juice.

After 2 to 3 hours, have her test the child's urine for glucose by mixing 2 drops of urine to 10 drops of water and 1 Clinitest tablet. Read after 15 seconds, comparing with color-coded card. (If card is not available from salesman, have her use 5 drops of urine to 10 drops of water and 1 Clinitest tablet. Read after 15 seconds, comparing with color code on paper supplied with Clinitest tablet.)

If this carbohydrate load gives the child a positive urine test, the parents should ask the family doctor for additional studies or referral to a diabetes clinic.

If a reagent tape, such as Chemstrip or Dextrostix, is used, about 1 hour after the cola have her test the child's blood (obtained with a fingerstick) by letting a drop fall on the tape. If the blood glucose level is over 165 mg/dl, the child should see the doctor.

Urine testing

Urine testing is easily taught. Still, mistakes are possible, so children should be supervised at least once or twice a week to be sure their technique is correct.

We teach them to use the 2-drop Clinitest, the most accurate urine glucose-testing method available, and to test for acetone during illness or high sugar spills with Acetest or Ketostix.

Blood glucose testing

We recommend blood glucose self-monitoring (BGSM) for young children as well as adolescents and adults. This testing technique provides more accurate information for insulin dosage modification. A variety of fingersticking devices, reagent tapes, and reflectance photometers are currently available. Regardless of the product your patient uses, we urge him to test his blood glucose levels four times a day every day during regulation and then four times a day 2 to 3 days a week when he's stable. We consider ideal testing times to be before breakfast (fasting), 2 hours before or after each meal, and at bedtime.

Insulin

The family may have trouble realizing at first that the twice-daily insulin shot will become as routine as brushing one's teeth. Anyone nervous about the use of the needle can practice on an orange, and indeed the child should. Sometimes to gain a child's confidence, we give the *parent* a "good" injection in front of him and then have the parent use the needle on the nurse. Once parents have given the *nurse* an injection, with a little practice they can give their child his injection, and he will trust them to. To overcome their fears, we encourage parents to remember they are giving a life-giving medicine.

The younger the child, the longer he will need to learn how to give himself his own shot. Practicing with an orange or a doll helps him work up his courage. Even then, he will probably cautiously try to work the needle through the skin rather than throw it in. But just teach him the basic procedure, and don't pressure him. Soon he will probably ask to give his own medication. We find that imitating his peers in the hospital is one of the strongest motivations. Warn the parents, however, that sooner or later he will give himself an uncomfortable shot at home. Unless they support him he may not want to give himself more for a long time.

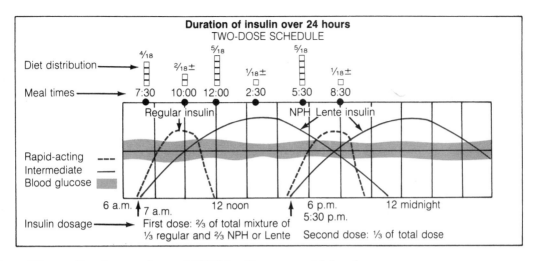

Duration of insulin over 24 hours
TWO-DOSE SCHEDULE

We usually give regular and NPH insulin — two thirds of the total insulin requirement in the morning, one third at night. One part of rapid-acting regular insulin along with two parts of the intermediate NPH insulin are given first thing in the morning, half an hour before breakfast; the remaining one third of the dose is given in equal parts of NPH and regular or, in smaller children, in the same proportion as in the morning, an hour before dinner (see chart above).

Refinements of the injection technique: equalizing pressure in both bottles by adding or withdrawing air before drawing the insulin into the syringe; always removing insulin from the same bottle first so that only one bottle will be adulterated by the other, if at all. Because children are so small, an air bubble can displace a significant amount of their daily insulin dose. Show the parents how to invert the syringe so gravity will get the bubbles out. Above all, work out a rotation pattern with them so that the same site will not be injected for at least a couple of weeks. Use a ½″ to ⅝″ needle so it will penetrate the skin and no further.

If the child shows a patterned sugar spill or elevated blood glucose level with BGSM at the same time each day, teach parents how to change timing of food or insulin or increase insulin. Infrequent or irregular spills need no change; frequent, regular spills need increased insulin or changed diet.

Insulin shock
Every parent must be prepared to recognize the first signs of hypoglycemia. Actually, each child seems to feel a little different from every other. The goal is to get him out of it

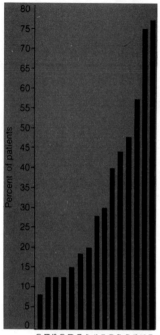

Onset symptoms

Marked onset, quick recognition
Onset symptoms of diabetes appear more frequently and more markedly in children than in adults. As a result, the disease tends to be diagnosed more quickly in children. In the above chart, the results of a study of 513 children with diabetes, you'll see that increased urination and thirst are common symptoms.

without starting, through overtreatment, the roller coaster effect we have described. Usually a 40- to 80-calorie increase in food is all that is needed; 1½ to 3 oz of juice or honey will do it rapidly. For mild to moderate reactions, glucose tablets, paste, or gel is preferred. If the reaction is severe, we recommend giving glucagon — which usually takes 15 to 20 minutes to work. In the hospital, 50% glucose is the drug choice.

In hypoglycemia, convulsions can occur. Parents should be ready to support their child in such an emergency. To warn parents of this possibility will add to their concern — but if they are prepared for it, the child will be in safer hands.

Diet management
In all three regimens for insulin administration — the four-dose per day, three-dose per day, and two-dose per day schedules — the child's calories should be distributed to give him one third in the morning, one third in the afternoon, and one third in the evening. To accommodate differences in rapid-acting and intermediate insulins, however, we calculate diets in terms of $\frac{1}{18}$ of the total calories.

Children at home usually receive insulin in two doses in the split-and-mix regimen. One dose, given ½ hour before breakfast, constitutes two thirds of the daily dose. It's a mixture of two parts of intermediate insulin and one part of rapid-acting insulin. The other dose (one third of the total daily dose) is given ½ hour before supper, and it's usually a 2:1 or 1:1 mixture of intermediate and rapid-acting insulin.

To accommodate the varying peak action of the insulin, the child should have his food distributed throughout the day with variation in this distribution related to increased or decreased exercise.

The usual pattern includes $\frac{4}{18}$ of the total daily calories for breakfast, ½ hour after the morning injection. The child should eat $\frac{1}{18}$ of the total daily calories 2 hours after breakfast. Then, he should eat $\frac{5}{18}$ for lunch and $\frac{2}{18}$ in midafternoon. Finally, he should eat $\frac{5}{18}$ for supper and $\frac{1}{18}$ at bedtime. The heavy afternoon snack could be "traded" for the morning or evening snack if increased activity usually occurs at those times. If the exercise pattern differs because of an unusual activity, food over and above the usual dietary plan could be added (or deleted), preferably before the activity (or rest).

The pattern, of course, also conforms generally to that of

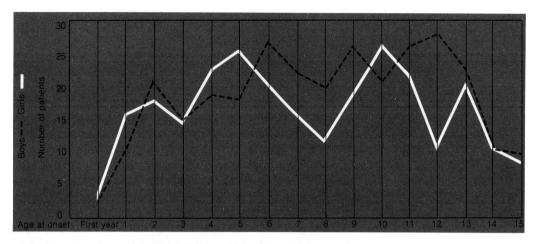

normal, active, nondiabetic children. They have higher metabolic needs than adults due to their growth. But with proportionately smaller stomachs, they best tolerate three meals and three between-meal snacks. As any mother of a normal adolescent will tell you, there's no other way to keep him satisfied.

During early childhood or the prepubescent growth spurt (or with retarded growth), the child needs 1.5 g of protein and 60 to 70 calories/kg of ideal weight per day. We advise parents closely on composition of this diet and give them instruction manuals.

Some diabetic diets involve measurements, but we find weighing food easier. It helps train the patient's eye for accurate proportioning. After having weighed food, children can eventually become skilled enough to estimate when they pass through a cafeteria line or are in situations where weighing is not practical. Thus skilled, they can feel freer to travel and choose their own foods. One precaution: The eye tends to "expand" a size, so it pays for parents and child to recheck weights every week or so.

Problems

One of the greatest difficulties will come in relating diet to exercise. If any child is abnormally active, he will need more food. But the child with diabetes uses glucose after exercise with less dependence on insulin. Therefore, he must have extra food, preferably *before* and *during* extra activity. Trial and error must determine if it is the right amount, judged by whether glucose is spilled in the urine, blood glucose level is elevated, or symptoms of hypoglycemia develop.

Age at onset
In children, the average age of diabetes onset seems to be 8 years, according to a study of 600 Type I diabetic patients. Diabetes occurs as often in boys as in girls.

We encourage parents to work toward two goals: when the child is well, to keep his urine as free of glucose and his blood glucose levels as near normal as possible without his experiencing an insulin reaction; when he is ill, to keep his urine glucose level down to less than 2% and free of acetone, and to keep his blood glucose levels as near normal as possible. Everything is recorded: urine or blood tests; the times, kinds, and amounts of the insulin injections; reactions; diet changes; and exercise. When accurate records are kept, danger signs are apparent. The doctor may have to increase the insulin whenever a cold or other infection strikes to keep it from making the child needlessly ill. Parents should know when to call.

Money is usually a problem in any chronic illness. If the parents know beforehand how much supplies and insulin cost, they will start to budget for future needs. Most of all, the child should be hospitalized long enough for him and his parents to be really well trained in managing his illness. A number of studies have determined that the more parents and families know about handling diabetes, the less hospitalization is needed later on. Perhaps this first time will be the only hospitalization a child will ever have for his metabolic flaw.

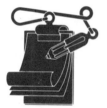

Remember these important points about diabetic children:
1. **Realize that a child with diabetes should receive insulin as soon as he is diagnosed.**
2. **Instruct the diabetic child and his family in the proper techniques for urine and blood glucose testing.**
3. **Be sure the family members of the diabetic child know how to recognize the first signs of hypoglycemia and are aware that, in most cases, a 40- to 80-calorie increase in food is all that's needed to correct it.**
4. **Accommodate the varying peaks of insulin by recommending that the diabetic child have his food distributed throughout the day with variations related to increased or decreased exercise.**
5. **When a diabetic child is well, encourage the parents to work toward this goal: Keep the child's urine glucose level down to less than 2% and his blood glucose levels as close to normal as possible without causing an insulin reaction.**

15

Pregnant diabetics:
Dispelling myths

BY CATHERINE GAROFANO, RN, BS

CONTEMPLATING MOTHERHOOD can be worrisome for any woman — especially if she lacks adequate prenatal instruction. For the diabetic patient, it's doubly so. That's why it's so important that all nurses who work with pregnant diabetic patients understand their unique problems.

Like most other women, a diabetic patient may be concerned about her emotional fitness for motherhood. But unlike most other women, she'll probably be more concerned about her *physical* fitness. Can she conceive? Would pregnancy adversely affect her diabetes? Would her diabetes harm her baby?

Confronted with these enormous concerns, she may turn to you with the unsettling question: "Should I have a baby?" Of course, you can't and shouldn't answer that question for her. But by separating the myths about diabetic pregnancy from the realities, you can help her and her husband answer it themselves.

Following are some common concerns and helpful answers. Before you get into these, read the chart on page 169. It explains diabetes-specialist Dr. Priscilla White's classification of diabetes according to onset and severity of disease. This widely used classification system will help you advise a diabetic woman on what complications, both fetal and maternal, she can anticipate during pregnancy.

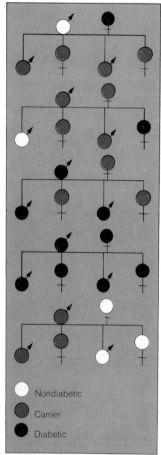

Nondiabetic

Carrier

Diabetic

Will your patient's child have diabetes?
Based on Mendelian statistics, the chances of a child developing diabetes would be as shown above. But these statistics are still indefinite since no one knows the exact relationship between heredity and diabetes. Recent studies suggest that the genetic factor is lower than once thought.

"Will I have trouble getting pregnant?"

Before insulin became available, the answer would have been an unqualified "yes." Few Type I diabetic patients lived to adulthood; many of those who did were sterile. Today, though, the answer is almost always "no." Usually only the most severely diabetic women or those with uncontrolled diabetes have trouble getting pregnant.

"Would I transmit diabetes to my baby?"

While it's true that diabetes has some genetic component, the risk of transmittal isn't as great as once thought. In fact, some statistics suggest that the child of a diabetic parent has as little as a 1% chance of developing diabetes before age 10. The risk increases with age. But the same statistics suggest that, even at age 60, the offspring of a diabetic parent still has only a 10% chance of developing diabetes. These percentages apply whether the mother or father is diabetic. If both are diabetic, though, the percentages double.

"Would the baby have more problems than the child of a healthy mother?"

Perhaps. Babies of diabetic mothers tend to be heavier, often more than 9 lb — especially if the mother develops diabetes during pregnancy (gestational diabetes) or is a Class A or Class B diabetic patient (as defined in the chart on the opposite page). Despite their heavy birth weight, they tend to be immature and are more likely to develop respiratory distress syndrome. Fortunately, though, this complication has been waning recently due to the development of indices that allow the doctor to select the best time for delivery.

Babies of diabetic fathers don't run any greater risk of congenital anomalies than babies of healthy parents. But babies of diabetic mothers run twice the risk (about 13% compared with 6% for the general population). Cardiac malformations, brain damage due to cerebral hemorrhage, traumatic birth due to the baby's large size, hypocalcemia or hyperbilirubinemia, and hypoglycemia are among the possible anomalies. Hypoglycemia used to be a common cause of neonatal death, but today, doctors can recognize it early and treat it promptly with glucose infusions. Today, the percentage of neonatal deaths among diabetic women who maintain normal blood glucose levels throughout their pregnancies is about the same as for

White's Classification of Pregnancy	
CLASS	DESCRIPTION
A	Abnormal glucose tolerance; no symptomatology; treated with diet only
B	Onset after age 19; duration of less than 10 years; no angiopathy
C	Diabetes of 10 to 19 years duration or onset between ages 10 and 19; no angiopathy
D	Diabetes of more than 20 years duration with onset before age 10 or with early angiopathy, background retinopathy, or calcified vessels in legs and feet
E	Pelvic vascular disease
F	Clinical evidence of nephropathy
R	Proliferative retinopathy
RF	Renal disease and proliferative retinopathy
G	Multiple abortions for stillbirths
H	Arteriosclerotic heart disease
T	Renal transplantation

the general population.

"Would I have more trouble with pregnancy than a non-diabetic woman? Would pregnancy make my diabetes worse?"

The effects of pregnancy all depend on the mother's condition. Pregnancy itself is an insulin-antagonistic state. That means a woman needs more insulin to maintain normal carbohydrate metabolism during pregnancy. A healthy person can meet that demand easily, but a woman with diabetes or a tendency toward diabetes can't. Her carbohydrate metabolism deteriorates, resulting in mild to severe hyperglycemia and even ketoacidosis if not adequately treated with insulin. Her blood glucose level should be maintained at 65 to 120 mg/dl.

Pregnant diabetic patients are more likely than nondiabetic patients to suffer from the following: hydramnios, toxemia, and urinary tract infections. Hydramnios, an excess of amniotic fluid, appears to some degree in about 20% of all pregnant diabetic patients. With judicious use of diuretics, though, doctors can prevent hydramnios from prematurely rupturing membranes. Diabetic patients also are five times more prone to toxemia with proteinuria, hypertension, and edema than the general population. There is an increased incidence of urinary tract infections that may adversely affect pregnancy. But these urinary tract infections usually respond quite well to medical therapy.

"Would I go into labor normally and deliver vaginally? Or would I deliver early, or would it be necessary for me to have a cesarean section?"

That depends on the mother's type of diabetes, her condition during pregnancy, and the baby's condition.

Incidence of Complications During Pregnancy by Diabetic Class

COMPLICATION	A	B	C	D	F	R
Spontaneous abortion rate	N	N	N	+	+ + + +	+ + + +
Hydramnios degree	+	+ + + +	+ + +	+ +	±	±
Excessive maternal weight gain	+	+ + + +	+ + +	+ +	0	0
Toxemia, i.e., preeclampsia	+	+ + + +	+ + +	+ +	?	Superimposed
Large placenta	+ + +	+ + + +	+ + +	+ +	0	0
Heavy-birth-weight infant	+ + + +	+ + + +	+ + +	+ +	0	0
Intrauterine fetal loss	+	+ +	+	+ + +	+ + + +	+ + + +
Intrapartum fetal loss	+ + + +	+ + + +	+ +	+	+	+
Neonatal loss	+	+	+ +	+ + +	+ + + +	+ + + +
Congenital abnormalities	+	+	+	+	+ +	+ + +
Diabetes mellitus intensified	+	+ + + +	+ + +	+	±	±

Key: N — normal; + — minimal chance; + + + + — maximum chance; 0 — not significant; ? — hard to tell; Superimposed — patient already had symptoms that are possibly made worse; ± — condition is possible

Rating the risks

The chart above details complications that may occur during a diabetic patient's pregnancy. The chances for each of these complications occurring are rated according to diabetic class (see White's pregnancy classification chart on the previous page). For example: A class B diabetic patient has a maximum chance for an intrapartum fetal loss. Refer to the chart's key to interpret the symbols.

If a woman is a Class A diabetic, the doctor will check her condition and the baby's size often, especially 1 week before the expected due date. If everything seems okay, he may allow her to go into spontaneous labor with a normal vaginal delivery. If he has any question about the expected delivery date, he'll usually induce labor somewhere during the 38th, 39th, or 40th week for a normal vaginal delivery. If pregnancy runs beyond the 40th week, he'll induce labor.

If a woman is a Class B or C diabetic, the doctor probably will induce labor during the 36th or 37th week. If she's a Class D, F, or R diabetic, he'll probably hospitalize her 6 to 8 weeks before her expected due date. And unless she needs an emergency delivery at some earlier time, he'll induce labor during the 35th or 36th week. In every case, he'll order chemical tests to determine the very best time for delivery.

If at all possible, most doctors prefer a vaginal delivery. But if the mother runs into complications, if the fetus shows signs of distress, or if the fetus is too large for an easy vaginal delivery, the doctor will perform a cesarean section.

"You said the doctor will determine the best time for delivery. How can he do that?"

With the help of a few simple tests.

First, he'll check the estriol level in the mother's urine or blood. A decrease in the estriol level indicates a failing placenta and may signal the need for immediate delivery. If the woman is a Class A, B, or C diabetic, the doctor will probably check her estriol level weekly, or more often after her 30th week of pregnancy.

Second, the doctor will monitor the baby's heart rate. A slowing heart rate indicates fetal distress and may mean it's time for immediate delivery. He'll also order several ultrasounds to monitor fetal growth.

If the ultrasounds are normal and the estriol level and fetal heart rate stay stable in the third trimester, the doctor will perform an amniocentesis and check the L/S ratio about the 36th or 37th week. The L/S ratio will help him pinpoint the best time for delivery.

"What exactly is the L/S ratio?"

The L/S, or lecithin/sphingomyelin, ratio is an analysis of lung phospholipids in the amniotic fluid, which is an index of fetal lung maturity. One of the main dangers of delivering a baby prematurely is the development of respiratory distress syndrome. When the L/S ratio reaches 2:1, the baby has much less chance of developing respiratory syndrome.

The test the L/S level, the doctor will obtain a sample of the amniotic fluid by aspirating it through the mother's abdomen.

"I get the impression I'll need a lot of medical attention during pregnancy. How often should I see my doctor?"

If a diabetic patient has reason to believe that she's pregnant, she should see her doctor as soon as possible. He'll do a thorough examination, including routine laboratory work and a complete history of her diabetes, to determine what class diabetic she is. In most cases, an obstetrician and an internist will see her every 2 weeks for the first and second trimester and once a week for the third trimester. At each appointment, they'll check her weight, blood pressure, blood glucose level, and urine and examine her for signs of hydramnios and edema. They'll also check the fundus of her eyes frequently. They'll

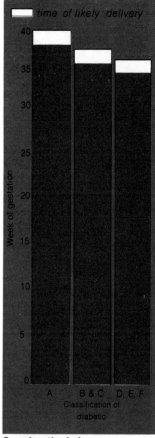

Carrying the baby
The more severe the mother's diabetes, the sooner doctors advise inducing labor to protect the health of mother and child.

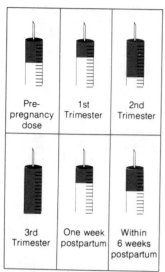

Pre-pregnancy dose	1st Trimester	2nd Trimester
3rd Trimester	One week postpartum	Within 6 weeks postpartum

Insulin needs during pregnancy
During the first trimester of pregnancy, insulin needs usually fall by one third. In fact, hypoglycemic reactions can be the first indication of pregnancy.

In the second trimester, insulin requirements rise to 66% above the prepregnancy dose, and by the last trimester, the patient's need for insulin rises to twice the prepregnancy dosage.

For about 5 days or so after delivery, most mothers have a temporary remission in their diabetes. Their need for insulin drops dramatically to about two thirds their prepregnancy dose. But within 6 weeks, they generally return to their normal insulin dosage.

evaluate her diabetic control and make any necessary changes in her diet or medication.

Just before the birth of her baby, a diabetic patient should contact a pediatrician to be present during delivery. Most babies do well during delivery, but a pediatrician should be on hand to handle any problems that might arise.

"Will I be able to take oral hypoglycemic agents during pregnancy?"

Most authorities don't recommend it. Oral hypoglycemic agents may not adequately control hyperglycemia, which could harm the baby. Also, the sulfonylureas (such as tolbutamide, chlorpropamide, glyburide, and glipizide) cross the placental barrier and enter the fetal circulation, which may cause prolonged hypoglycemia and possibly fetal death. If a woman is taking oral hypoglycemic agents before pregnancy, her doctor will probably switch her to insulin during her pregnancy.

"Will my insulin requirements change during pregnancy?"

Yes. In fact, they'll probably fluctuate. Insulin requirements frequently decrease during the first trimester. This effect isn't completely understood but may be due to the utilization of glucose by the fetoplacental unit. Insulin requirements usually increase during the second and third trimesters, due to the insulin-antagonist state that results primarily from the placenta's production of hormones, such as estrogen, progesterone, and lactogen, as the placenta enlarges. It also results from a slight elevation in the free T_4 (thyroxine) and a slight increase in an adrenal cortical hormone known as cortisol. An insulin-degrading enzyme in the placenta, known as insulinase, also may increase the insulin requirement. Decreased insulin requirements during the second and third trimesters may indicate a failing placenta.

"What about my diet? Should I stick to it during pregnancy?"

Yes, but with a few slight changes to ensure that the mother and her baby get all the nutrients they need.

During pregnancy, a diabetic diet is modified to increase the carbohydrate intake. Severe restriction of carbohydrate could predispose a pregnant diabetic patient to ketosis, which could harm her baby. To supply the baby with enough nutrition, the total daily caloric requirement is about 30 calories/kg of ideal body weight. If she's overweight, she may need to reduce her weight during pregnancy, but she shouldn't eat any less than 1,400 calories/day.

A pregnant diabetic patient also should have a protein intake of about 1½ or 2 g/kg of ideal body weight. And she should keep fat intake stable. Since excess weight will predispose her to toxemia, she should keep her weight gain to 25 lb or less.

"Should I keep testing my urine for glucose and ketones?"
Yes, if this is the monitoring method the doctor selects. In this instance, a pregnant diabetic patient should keep checking a urine specimen for glucose and ketones before meals and in the evening before bedtime. If urine glucose stays at 1% to 2% for more than three or four consecutive tests, she should report this to her doctor. If she gets a positive ketone reading, with or without glucose, she should report it to her doctor immediately. Ketones *without* glucose usually mean that the woman isn't taking enough carbohydrates. Ketones *with* glucose often herald the onset of ketoacidosis, which could cause fetal death in the second half of pregnancy.

During lactation, Benedict's and Clinitest urine glucose tests will be totally unreliable. That's because lactose, or milk sugar, spills into urine, giving high positive readings on these tests. During lactation, a diabetic can use Tes-Tape since it tests glucose specifically. Still, as a rapid-testing method, it will indicate only a range of concentration rather than an absolute value. Remember that pregnancy creates a low renal threshold for glucose. A pregnant diabetic patient also should have frequent blood glucose analyses.

Many doctors advocate blood glucose self-monitoring (BGSM) at home instead of, or along with, urine testing. A pregnant patient should check her blood glucose level 6 to 10 times daily. If she gets a blood glucose reading above 120 mg/dl, she should report it to her doctor immediately.

"How would my insulin requirement be handled during delivery?"
Most likely the doctor will admit a pregnant diabetic patient to the hospital a few days before delivery to ensure maximum control of her diabetes before and during delivery. On the day

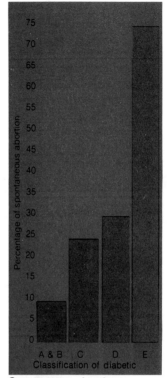

Spontaneous abortions
Expectant diabetic patients sometimes worry that their diabetes will prevent them from carrying their babies to term. Reassure them that the risk of spontaneous abortion is far smaller than it once was. Of course, the more severe an expectant mother's diabetes is, the greater a risk she runs of losing her child. In all but the most severe diabetic patients, though, chance of delivery far outweighs chance of spontaneous abortion.

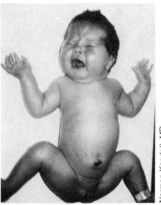

A matter of size
This baby's mother is a diabetic patient; as a result, at birth the baby weighed 9 lb 11 oz, large for her gestational age. Class A and B diabetics, as well as mothers who develop diabetes during pregnancy, often have heavy babies even though many are born prematurely. These babies lose the excess weight, largely due to fluid, shortly after birth.

of delivery, he'll cut her intermediate insulin dosage in half. Then, he'll restrict food and fluids by mouth and start an intravenous infusion of dextrose 5% in water at a rate of 1,000 ml every 8 hours until the patient has delivered.

The doctor will have blood glucose level testing done every 4 to 6 hours and elevations covered with regular insulin.

At the time of delivery, and usually for 48 to 72 hours afterwards, insulin requirements drop dramatically to the point where insulin may not be needed at all. During this period, the mother should be watched closely for signs of hypoglycemia. Her insulin requirements will return to the prepregnancy state within a week. If she has gestational diabetes, she may not need insulin after delivery at all.

"Will I be able to breast-feed my baby?"
Yes. The only caution is that a diabetic mother remain on insulin if she's been taking oral hypoglycemic agents prior to the pregnancy. Studies have confirmed that oral hypoglycemic agents get into the milk of lactating women. They haven't confirmed any adverse effect on nursing babies yet, but hypoglycemia in the infant is a possibility. To be on the safe side, a diabetic mother probably shouldn't take them if she's nursing her baby.

Because of nurses' expanding role, you have the good fortune to serve as patient counselor and instructor in diabetology, family planning, and prenatal and postnatal care. As an important member of the medical team, you can help ensure optimum success for your pregnant diabetic patient.

Remember these important points concerning pregnancy in a patient with diabetes:
1. **Keep in mind that the risk of a diabetic mother transmitting diabetes to her child is relatively low.**
2. **Realize that babies of diabetic mothers who maintain normal blood glucose levels throughout pregnancy don't run any greater risk of congenital anomalies than babies of nondiabetic mothers.**
3. **Inform your diabetic patient that if she's taking oral hypoglycemic agents prior to pregnancy, her doctor will probably switch her to insulin during pregnancy.**
4. **If your diabetic patient has taken oral hypoglycemic agents prior to pregnancy, assure her that she will be able to breast-feed her baby as long as she remains on insulin.**

16

Blind diabetics:
Breeding independence

BY JOYCE SCHULZ, RN, AND
MARIE WILLIAMS, BA, MSW

WHY TRY TO make a blind diabetic patient independent? Isn't it easier just to make sure that his family, friends, or clinic will premeasure his insulin and test his urine or blood glucose? In fact, isn't it safer?

Yes, management by others is easier and maybe a little safer. And some blind diabetic patients may prefer it. But most blind diabetic patients, even those with supportive spouses, crave independence. And nearly all but the most severely diabetic patients could achieve it *if encouraged to.* Unfortunately, though, few health professionals give that encouragement. Too many of them feel that treatment should aim at absolute control with no risks. As well-meaning as that goal is, it overlooks the chief concern of many blind diabetic patients: a fulfilling life with minimal dependence on sighted persons. The health professionals' fears also reinforce those of the patient.

In our experience at the Minneapolis Society for the Blind, working primarily with diabetic patients, we've come to feel that you can't work adequately with a blind diabetic patient unless you understand the emotional impact of his blindness. You also need to understand the effect of blindness on diabetic control and the practical skills that the patient can learn to control his condition.

A double blow

Blindness comes as a tremendous shock to anyone, even an otherwise healthy person or someone whose vision has been fading for years. Suddenly the blind person realizes that he can't do all those things that we take for granted in everyday life — reading, writing, applying cosmetics, shaving, working, even just walking around freely. Since all of these activities are tied to our sense of self-worth, the most common reaction of any newly blind person is to feel that he's lost his worth as a person. He's still the person he was before, with all the same needs and goals. But to live a normal life, he has to start from scratch and relearn even the simplest activity.

Still, if blindness is a person's only handicap, he can usually master new techniques — traveling with a cane or dog, for instance; reading in braille; typing instead of writing; using special devices to cook, keep house, work.

For the diabetic patient, though, blindness comes as a double blow. Because of related health difficulties — loss of tactile sensitivity, for instance, or circulatory impairment — he may have more difficulty using braille, moving around well, or keeping up with a job. Worst of all, blindness interferes with two activities essential to his very existence: giving himself insulin injections and testing his urine or blood glucose. Still, most blind diabetic patients want these skills so much that their desire often outweighs any difficulties.

Unfounded concerns about injections

Our experience indicates that, contrary to the assumption of some health professionals and patients, self-management of diabetes by blind patients needn't be dangerous or impossible. Of the more than 300 blind diabetic patients we've worked with, only a very few of those who wanted to become independent failed to learn how to measure and inject their insulin.

Many professionals and patients voice two concerns about self-injections: first, that the patient might inject a dangerous amount of air into subcutaneous tissue and, second, that he'll make a dangerous injection into a blood vessel. Let us lay both concerns to rest.

If a patient is taught proper techniques, he can't inject more than a harmlessly tiny amount of air into subcutaneous tissue. The only real danger to guard against is getting an air bubble so large that it displaces a significant quantity of insulin. By

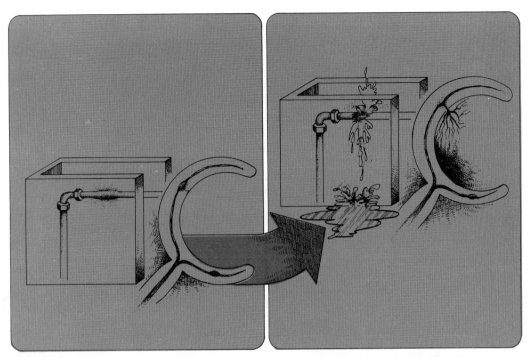

slowly withdrawing and reinjecting insulin into the vial three times before the actual injection and by holding the vial perpendicular to keep the insulin level, though, he can eliminate any large bubbles.

If the patient uses prescribed injection sites and techniques, he also runs little risk of injecting into a blood vessel — even though he won't be able to pull back the plunger to check for blood.

To make insulin injections as risk-free as possible, we also teach the following precautions:

• When giving himself an injection, the patient should stabilize his hand by placing his little finger against the skin and using it to locate the injection site. He then should gently insert the needle through the skin rather than use the more common dartlike motion. (Of course, there's no need to pull back on the plunger.)

• The patient must keep an accurate record of how many doses he's used so he'll know when his bottle is empty. One method of keeping an accurate record involves putting as many marbles as doses in a container and removing one marble after each injection. To keep the insulin level from getting too low, he should throw the bottle away when two doses remain.

Like a leaky pipe
In background retinopathy (illustrated above left), blood vessel abnormalities are contained within the retina. Proliferative retinopathy (illustrated above right) is a more serious problem. Blood vessels hemorrhage through the retina surface into the vitreous, like a leaky pipe breaking through a wall.

Special equipment for the vision-impaired diabetic

Before beginning your teaching sessions with a diabetic patient, find out if he has impaired vision. Because many patients won't admit that they have trouble seeing, this can hinder your teaching efforts and jeopardize the therapy's effectiveness. Some of the devices available for the visually impaired or blind diabetic patient are shown here.

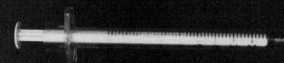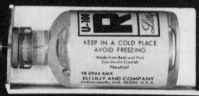

AFB needle guide

This metal guide, shown here, is custom-cut to accommodate any size insulin bottle. The following instructions explain how to use it: Place the needle in the V-shaped notch. Then, lay the bottle in the trough so the stopper faces the notch. Push the bottle along the trough to insert the needle into the stopper.

Remember, once the notch is cut, this guide can only be used with one size bottle. Also, when this device is used, the needle can easily become contaminated.

Dos-Aid Syringe Filling Device

This plastic device accommodates disposable U-100 syringes. The doctor will position the plunger stop at a point determined by the dose. Then he'll tighten the stop so it can't be moved, thereby governing the amount of insulin drawn up each time by the patient.

The Dos-Aid Syringe Filling Device has these disadvantages: the needle can become easily contaminated, and the plunger stop may loosen and move with repeated use.

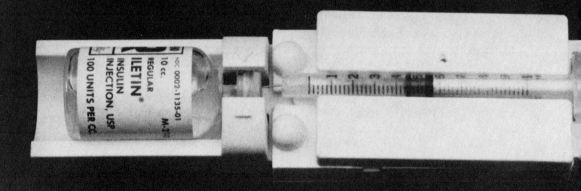

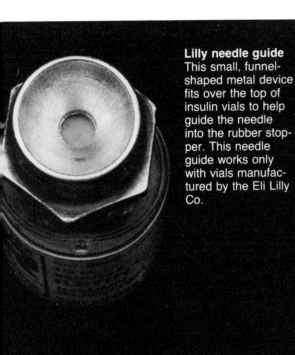

Lilly needle guide
This small, funnel-shaped metal device fits over the top of insulin vials to help guide the needle into the rubber stopper. This needle guide works only with vials manufactured by the Eli Lilly Co.

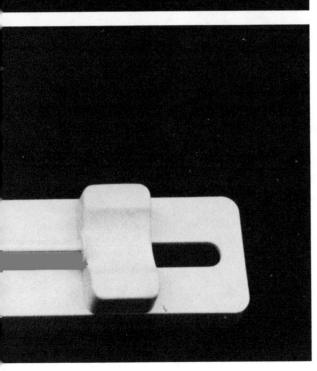

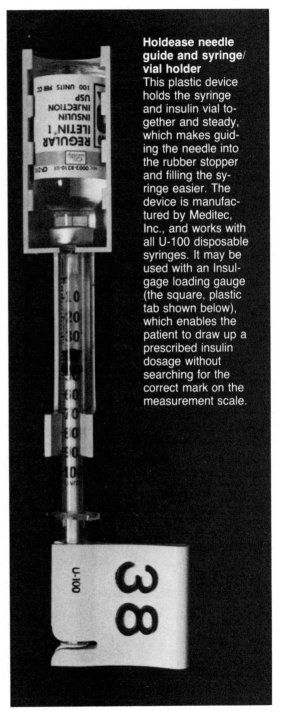

Holdease needle guide and syringe/vial holder
This plastic device holds the syringe and insulin vial together and steady, which makes guiding the needle into the rubber stopper and filling the syringe easier. The device is manufactured by Meditec, Inc., and works with all U-100 disposable syringes. It may be used with an Insulgage loading gauge (the square, plastic tab shown below), which enables the patient to draw up a prescribed insulin dosage without searching for the correct mark on the measurement scale.

A stick in time

Blind diabetic patients may test their blood glucose levels themselves at home by putting a drop of their blood on a reagent strip. Patients can choose from these five devices: the Autoclix (Bio-Dynamics), the Autolet (Owen Mumford, distributed by Ulster Scientific), the Hemalet (Medprobe), the Penlet (Lifescan), and the Monojector (Monoject Division, Sherwood Medical). The photos at right show you how to use three of these devices. Before using the bloodletting device, have the patient choose a puncture site. Tell him to wash his hands or clean the site with alcohol. Then, instruct him to squeeze his fingertip.

Autoclix

If he's using the Autoclix, instruct him to insert a new Monolet lancet (Sherwood Medical) by depressing the plunger. Have him remove the protective cap and place the lancet at the puncture site. To push the lancet into the skin, have him gently push the Autoclix unit.

Autolet

Suppose the patient chooses to use the Autolet. Have him put on a new platform and insert a new Monolet. When he removes the protective cap, tell him to place the platform on the puncture site. To operate the arm containing the lancet, have him simply press the button.

Hemalet

Tell a patient using the Hemalet to begin by inserting a new Monolet and removing the protective cap. Have him place a guard over the lancet. Now instruct him to pull back on the Hemalet's cap until he feels it click into place. After he positions the guard at the puncture site, have him gently squeeze the red release bars together.

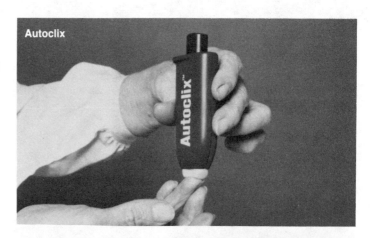

Autoclix

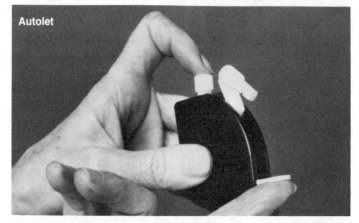

Autolet

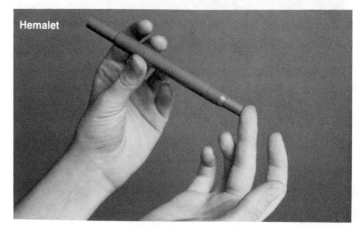

Hemalet

Glucose testing: Essential for insulin control

More than self-injections, self-testing of urine and blood poses a problem to blind diabetic patients. Science for the Blind manufactures an audible urine testing device that beeps in response to changes in Tes-Tape colors. For example, it sounds one beep for a negative test, two beeps for $\frac{1}{10}\%$, three beeps for $\frac{1}{4}\%$, and four beeps for $\frac{1}{2}\%$.

A well-motivated blind diabetic patient can perform blood glucose self-monitoring using reagent tapes. However, a sighted person must be available to ensure that the diabetic patient gets a drop of blood on the tape and to read the results. Recently, researchers developed an audible adaptor for the glucose monitoring device. Researchers are also working on a new fingerstick device that will ensure the blind diabetic patient gets an adequate drop of blood on the strip. When these devices are widely available, blind diabetic patients will finally have an equal opportunity to manage their own care.

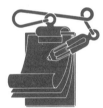

Remember these important points about promoting independence for blind diabetic patients:

1. Teach your patient how to eliminate large air bubbles during insulin injection by slowly withdrawing and reinjecting insulin into the vial three times before the actual injection. Remind him to hold the vial perpendicular.

2. Assure him that if he uses prescribed injection sites and techniques he runs little risk of injecting insulin into a blood vessel.

3. Advise your patient to insert the needle gently through the skin instead of using the more common dartlike motion.

4. To know when his insulin bottle is empty, have him keep an accurate record of how many doses he's used.

5. Familiarize yourself — and your patient — with special equipment for administering insulin and testing urine and blood glucose.

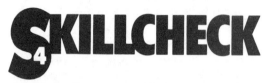

SKILLCHECK

1. Johnny Stover, age 12, is on a 2,600-calorie diet of three meals and three snacks. He also takes a split dose of insulin, one dose before breakfast and one before dinner. Johnny plays Little League baseball after school 3 days a week. What adjustments would you advise him to make on those days?

2. Several months ago, Mary Willis, age 2, was discovered to have diabetes when she was brought into the hospital with convulsive hypoglycemic reactions. Since then, Mrs. Willis has been terrified of a blood glucose level below 150 mg/dl. But she is trying to keep Mary on a strict routine that will keep her diabetes under complete control around the clock. How would you educate Mrs. Willis about Mary's diabetic condition?

3. Terry, age 15, is going through a trying adolescence. She is denying her diabetes and hiding it from her friends because "they wouldn't want to hang around with someone who's sick all the time." How could you help Terry develop a more positive outlook on her disease?

4. Debby Rosen developed diabetes at age 11. She is now 27 and wants to begin a family. However, she and her husband are concerned about pregnancy. Debby says she doesn't have any complications from her diabetes and she controls it well. But she's afraid pregnancy will make her diabetes worse. What would you tell her?

5. Ed Phillips is 44 years old. His visual acuity is: right eye, counting fingers at 1'; left eye, no light perception. Right now he is living with his brother, but in a few months he'll be living by himself in an apartment. Although he must move to be close to the radio station where he'll be working, Mr. Phillips is apprehensive about managing his diabetes alone. How would you prepare him for his move?

6. Eileen Shaunnessy, age 53, has managed her insulin injections well for nearly 10 years. Now, however, her sight is

failing and she has trouble making sure she's drawing up the right amount of insulin and eliminating air bubbles. What would you recommend?

7. Nancy Byers, who controls her diabetes with 100 mg Tolinase daily, has just learned that she's pregnant with her first child. She's delighted but concerned about taking her Tolinase during pregnancy. She's heard it will hurt the baby and says she's going to stop taking it. What would you tell her?

8. Ted Nichols, age 16, is on a daily dose of 8 units regular insulin and 28 units NPH. He's planning to go backpacking in the Rockies. Although Ted has always been active, a backpacking trip will be slightly more exerting than he's used to. How would you advise him to plan for his trip?

9. Susan Hendricks has delivered a 9-lb, 4-oz baby girl by cesarean section. She has decided to breast-feed her baby, which means she will continue taking insulin. On her first day home, Susan tests her blood glucose and gets a reading of 240 mg/dl. Very upset, she calls you and asks what to do. Should she take more insulin?

(Answers begin on page 207)

HOW TO GIVE IN-HOSPITAL CARE

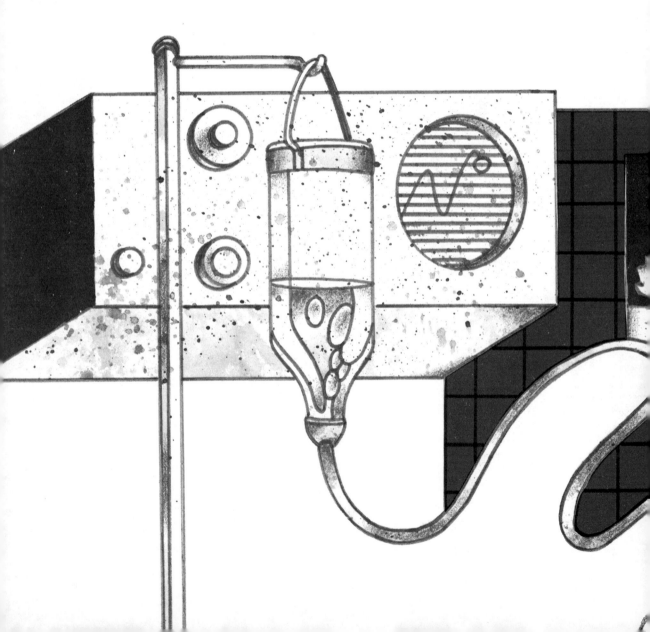

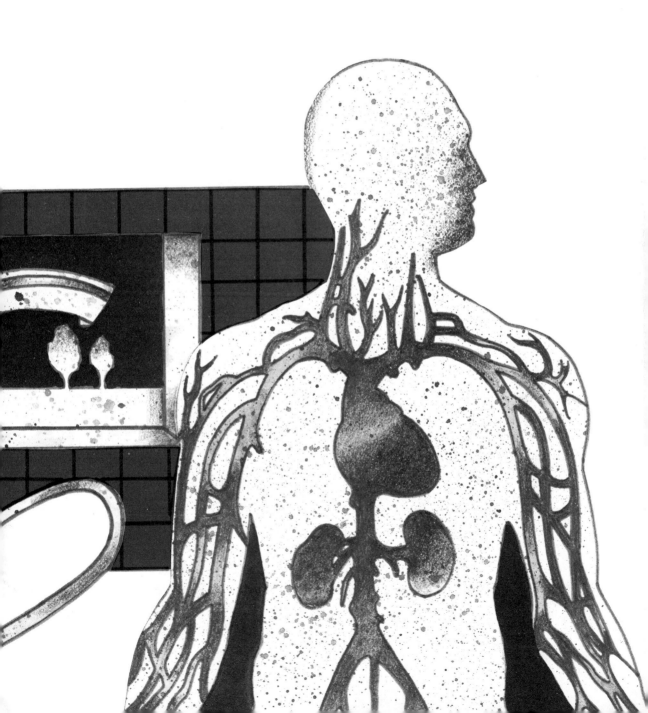

If your diabetic patient
is receiving nasogastric suction,
what nursing measures would you take
to help prevent acidosis, electrolyte
imbalance,
and dehydration?

What makes a diabetic patient
more prone to infection than a
nondiabetic patient?

If your diabetic patient
is recovering from surgery,
what life-threatening complications
might you expect to find?

What is the best time
to schedule diagnostic procedures
for an insulin-dependent
diabetic patient?

17

Skirting ill effects of surgery

BY EDWINA A. McCONNELL, RN, MS

SURGERY IS STRESS enough for the healthy patient. For the diabetic patient, it is even more critical. With his own metabolism already more or less balanced on a seesaw, where ketoacidosis could await him if he slips off to one side and insulin shock if he tilts too far to the other, he faces a special situation. Not only do illness, surgery, and convalescence interrupt his normal food intake, his eating schedule, and any insulin or medication program he may follow, but something else happens to intensify the effects of the interruption.

Normally, his regimen has been aimed at controlling his blood glucose levels on an everyday plane, but now stress releases adrenocorticotropic hormone (ACTH) from the pituitary. The ACTH stimulates the adrenal cortex to produce glucocorticoids. These hormones increase gluconeogenesis and the extra glucose goes directly into the bloodstream. Meantime, the catecholamine epinephrine, also normally released under stress to prepare the body for a fight or flight, spurs the conversion of stored glycogen to available glucose; this, too, raises the blood glucose levels. That calls for more insulin.

A typical case is Angela S., age 23, a magazine staff writer who was hospitalized for a cystoscopy because of recurrent microscopic amounts of blood in her urine. Angela had been diagnosed as having diabetes a year earlier.

Since then, she had followed a diet based on 1,500 calories; 150 g of it were carbohydrate, 75 g protein, and 75 g fat, a typical diabetic diet based on 15 calories to the pound of body weight with a ratio of 2:1:1 carbohydrate, protein, and fat, respectively. Angela's current insulin regimen was 20 units of Lente (intermediate) insulin and 10 units of Semilente (rapid-acting) insulin daily before breakfast.

Her blood glucose level was normally between 200 and 250 mg/dl. Once or twice during regulation she had reported preliminary symptoms of shock to her doctor. Yet the evening she was hospitalized, her blood glucose level was 350 mg/dl. But she gave no sign of an infection. We decided that the stress of anxiety was probably the culprit.

Angela S. was anxious about the next day's procedure and its possible revelation. She was quite worried about cancer, which ran in her family. All this anxiety was throwing her conscientiously regulated metabolism to the winds.

The problems of metabolic regulation we encountered with Angela are the essential ones faced by every diabetic patient undergoing surgery — and his doctor and his nurse. Such a patient needs a consistently stable internal environment. That means we need to:

• prevent severe fluid loss brought about through the osmotic diuresis forced by hyperglycemia

• prevent ketosis that would follow insulin deficiency

• prevent the diabetic coma that could follow ketoacidosis, *but also* ward off the opposite: hypoglycemia and insulin shock.

As a bonus, these steps also minimize the patient's predisposition to infection and spare his body any wasting of protein that he needs for tissue repair.

Just how you will do this depends, of course, on the doctor's preferences for treating diabetes. And it depends on other things, such as the type of diabetes and the presence of any diabetic complications. It also depends on any coexisting conditions and on the nature of the surgery.

As for type, the patient with Type II diabetes (usually someone much older than Angela) is likely to be on a diet or diet-and-oral agent regimen for control. He is usually able to tolerate the stress of either minor or major surgery with little metabolic disturbance — provided he has no infection. (Infection is one of the stresses that raises blood glucose levels.) In fact, he may be able to get through a minor procedure under a local anesthetic with little change in his daily management.

The Type I diabetic patient controls his diabetes with daily doses of intermediate insulin, sometimes in conjunction with regular (rapid-acting) insulin, as Angela's was controlled. He requires close observation and careful monitoring. The day of surgery he can usually be safely managed (if he has no infection) with an I.V. solution of dextrose 5% in water and the administration of rapid-acting insulin in amounts dictated by blood glucose determinations.

Insulin needs can also swing wildly when an occasional patient develops insulin resistance. In this, thousands of units bind with insulin antibodies. However, most patients with this problem ultimately require large doses of insulin — usually greater than 200 units/day.

As for the nature of surgery, the terms "minor" and "major" denote the total stresses associated with a surgical procedure. This means not only the extent of physical trauma involved (including that of organ manipulation and the amount of tissue incised and sutured), but also the length of time the operation takes, the anesthetic agent used, and — underlying it all, of course — the patient's psychological response. Major surgical procedures lasting several hours, such as radical mastectomy, thoracotomy, subtotal gastrectomy, or abdominal perineal resection, cause the greatest disruption in metabolic control. Minor procedures, such as cystoscopy, cataract removal, dilatation and curettage, and tooth extractions, cause the least. Certainly a cystoscopy was not exactly a major procedure — except to Angela S. and to anyone who could understand why she might be concerned.

Individualizing nursing care

Each patient is a unique human being with individual needs and ways of coping. The patient undergoing surgery, with or without diabetes, is indisputably no exception. Major or minor to you, the surgery will be major to him. Not only is his body the target of a planned assault, but his mind becomes a breeding ground for anxiety, conjecture, and concern. If you can work with the patient preoperatively, that may relieve some

Common diabetic conditions
No pathologic difference exists between the surgical conditions of diabetic patients and those of normal patients. But diabetic patients are more prone to several conditions that may require surgery. Among them: gallstones, cancer of the pancreas and general malignant disease, Dupuytren's contracture, soft tissue infection, and gangrene of the extremities.

of his anxiety and facilitate a smoother postoperative course. Assess each patient and, together with him, plan his care.

Preoperatively, he will probably need the following laboratory tests and studies: hemoglobin, complete blood count, blood urea nitrogen, creatinine, serum electrolytes, fasting blood glucose, p.m. blood glucose (if he's insulin-dependent), routine urinalysis with emphasis on glucose and ketone, EKG, and chest films.

He should also have blood glucose drawn at the same time his urine is tested for glucose and ketone. Why? Because most patients with Type II diabetes have high renal thresholds (200 to 300 mg/dl), their urine test results can be misleading. (When a nondiabetic patient's blood glucose ranges between 160 and 180 mg/dl, urine glucose test results will typically be positive.)

Most important, he should have blood glucose drawn 1 hour preoperatively. If the level is low, he's going to need a glucose infusion (dextrose 5% in water) to prevent hypoglycemia during surgery. But, regardless of the blood glucose results, *all* insulin-dependent diabetic patients should have an intravenous access throughout surgery in case any problems arise. Angela's blood glucose levels had been brought down to 150 mg/dl with 10 units of regular insulin just before surgery. Her doctors were satisfied to have a slight margin of reserve glucose on hand to ward off hypoglycemia, which can be dangerous and hard to detect in an unconscious patient.

For the usual diabetic patient, the dosage of preoperative morphine or meperidine will be reduced by one quarter or one half, because the nausea and vomiting that these drugs can all too easily cause will *decrease* his need for insulin, enhancing his chances of a hypoglycemic reaction. Infection and fever, unlike nausea and vomiting, are known to raise blood glucose levels.

Understanding methods of control

Doctors use numerous methods to keep the patient free of ketoacidosis and acetonuria, dehydration, and hypoglycemia and its shock. You must be familiar with the methods used and be acutely aware of the treatment course chosen for *your* patient. The decision on the best way to prepare a diabetic patient, especially a patient with Type I diabetes, for surgery usually depends on the doctor's preference and the patient's prescribed regimen. As a general guideline, here are several of the methods commonly used by specialists.

Diet-controlled Type II diabetes. This patient's doctor may decide to ensure stabilization by admitting the patient to the hospital 1 to 2 days before surgery; that way, dietary slip-ups can be prevented. On the day of surgery, a fasting blood glucose reading should be obtained: this reading serves as a baseline for subsequent blood glucose levels obtained later in the day. Throughout the patient's perioperative period, he should be observed for such complications as hyperglycemia, ketoacidosis, and hyperosmolar coma (a serious threat to elderly patients).

Oral agent–controlled Type II diabetes. If the patient controls his diabetes with an oral agent as well as diet, he'll probably also be admitted to the hospital 1 to 2 days before surgery. For most such patients, the usual oral agent dose is withheld before major surgery. For example, the oral agent chlorpropamide should be discontinued 36 hours before surgery, because that's the half-life of this agent. Remember, patients taking this oral agent should be closely observed for hypoglycemia during and after surgery because of the agent's long half-life. (Most other oral agents cause a less significant drop in blood glucose levels.)

When an oral agent is withheld, the patient's insulin needs are met by adding 10 units of regular insulin to a liter of dextrose 5% in water either during surgery or postoperatively. When a patient's postoperative blood glucose level is greater than 250 mg/dl, 10 units of regular insulin are given subcutaneously, and the regular insulin added to subsequent infusions is increased to 16 units.

For most patients, mixing regular insulin with the dextrose infusion poses no significant problems. Depending on the I.V. fluid container, insulin usually is stable in either 5% or 10% solutions of dextrose and water, with or without electrolytes. But this method has too many variables to be completely reliable; that's why many medical centers have replaced it with other methods.

You may think that simultaneous infusion of both dextrose solution and insulin would afford smoother control of the diabetes. Unfortunately, the opposite is true: this method usually gives poor dosage control and can produce fluctuations in the patient's blood glucose level. This is because, when insulin is administered in I.V. solutions, a large percentage of it may adhere to both the bottle and the tubing, meaning that the patient receives a greatly reduced and fluctuating dose. This problem may be prevented by adding several milliliters of the patient's blood to the dextrose solution.

Remember: If you must add insulin to the I.V., be sure it's regular. This will prevent delayed reactions.

If the patient who controls his diabetes with diet and an oral agent is undergoing minor surgery, continue this method to reserve a sulfonylurea for postoperative administration, as recommended. Replace each missed meal with 50 g of I.V. dextrose. If the patient can't tolerate his oral agent, titrate regular insulin according to his blood glucose level.

Type I diabetes. This patient is usually admitted to the hospital for monitoring 1 to 2 days before surgery. If his blood glucose levels are greater than 200 mg/dl, he should receive regular crystalline zinc insulin at frequent intervals along with (or in place of) his intermediate or long-acting insulin. He should have no signs or symptoms of hyperglycemia.

Obtain a fasting blood glucose reading the morning of surgery, and start an intravenous infusion of dextrose 5% in water or saline.

Unfortunately, no ideal method of control — one that would indicate the amount and type of insulin needed and the time it should be given — has been discovered. The following five methods are most commonly used:

• Many doctors follow the split–normal dose method, which is recommended by the American Diabetes Association. For the patient who can achieve daily control with intermediate insulin alone or combined with regular (rapid-acting) insulin, an I.V. infusion of dextrose 5% in water provides the necessary carbohydrates. Once the infusion has been started, a reduced dose of the usual insulin mixture — usually one half the normal maintenance dose — is given subcutaneously. The remainder of the usual dose is given subcutaneously in the recovery room or when the patient returns to his room after surgery.

This dosage method will avert the very serious threat of insulin shock during surgery.

Specialists feel that transient hyperglycemia would be far less harmful. But this method requires closer postoperative observation.

If the patient misses any meals, he should continue to receive an intravenous infusion of dextrose 5% in water or dextrose 5% in normal saline solution administered at a rate that provides 3,000 ml of fluid and 150 g of glucose through the 24-hour period.

• Another method of control substitutes regular insulin for the patient's usual intermediate or long-acting insulin. This method keeps his blood glucose levels more responsive to moment-by-moment control. Preoperatively, the patient should receive 1 unit of regular crystalline insulin for every 2 g of dextrose to be given, followed by insulin supplements.

• A third method of control substitutes four equal doses of regular insulin (given subcutaneously at 6-hour intervals on the day of surgery) for the patient's usual intermediate or long-acting insulin. To maintain and replace fluids, an adequate amount of dextrose 5% in one third normal saline solution is given preoperatively, Ringer's lactate is used during surgery, and one fourth to one half of a normal multiple electrolyte solution is given postoperatively. Keep in mind that if dextrose 5% doesn't adequately maintain the patient's blood glucose levels, a dextrose 10% solution can be used. Obtain urine or blood specimens to determine the necessary dosage of supplemental insulin.

To determine that dosage, fractional urines for glucose and ketone are used along with blood glucose determinations. But a word of caution: don't collect urine that's been sitting in the patient's bladder overnight or even for several hours, because it will tell more about the past than about the present so far as spilling glucose or ketone into the urine is concerned. Instead, test the second voided specimen.

To obtain a urine specimen from a patient with a Foley catheter, simply clamp the catheter for 15 to 30 minutes. Then, use the catheter's aspiration port to obtain the specimen. If the catheter does not have this port, *do not disconnect the catheter from its tubing*. Instead, clean the catheter with an alcohol wipe and aspirate a small amount of urine using a 25G needle to puncture the catheter.

But before testing the urine for glucose and ketone, note what medications the patient is getting. With Clinitest tablets, large quantities of ascorbic acid, NegGram, the cephalosporins, or probenecid can give false-positive readings. Yet, except for ascorbic acid, these medications have no effect on glucose testing done with Tes-Tape, Hema-Combistix, Com-

Using blood glucose levels to determine a sliding scale
Instead of using urine glucose levels to determine a sliding scale insulin dosage, some hospitals are using blood glucose levels. Sliding scales vary because each must be tailored to the individual patient's needs and his doctor's preference. Here's an example of one patient's sliding scale: If the patient's blood glucose level is 180 mg/dl, he receives no insulin; for 240 mg/dl, he receives 2 to 6 units; for 400 mg/dl, 5 to 16 units; and for 800 mg/dl, 13 to 16 units.

bistix, Uristix, Clinistix, Keto-Diastix, or Diastix.

For most patients, regular insulin is given by 5-unit increments in accordance with percentage increases on the reagent scale. For example, for a urine glucose level of 0 to 0.25%, the patient receives no insulin. For 0.5%, he receives 5 units; for 1%, 10 units; for 2%, 15 units. If he's acidotic, another 5 units may be given (For information on a sliding scale based on blood glucose levels, see information at left).

• Still another method of control for the patient with Type I diabetes uses the Biostator Glucose Monitor Controller. This commercially available closed-loop artificial pancreas controls blood glucose levels during and after surgery.

• Some doctors prefer to infuse regular insulin along with a separate infusion of dextrose and water. You can start these infusions preoperatively and continue them through and after surgery until the patient can take fluids orally. Usually 1 to 2 units of regular insulin and 5.0 to 7.5 g of glucose per hour are given by I.V. drip to maintain the patient's blood glucose level in the desired range of 150 to 250 mg/dl.

Prepare the insulin solution by adding 50 units of regular insulin to 500 ml of 0.9% sodium chloride. This insulin concentration of 1.0 units/10 ml is best managed using an infusion pump.

Insulin-induced hypoglycemia is a critical problem that, in many cases, occurs when the I.V. containing the glucose infiltrates. Manage this potential complication by carefully evaluating the patient's blood glucose levels as well as his clinical status.

Goals of postoperative care
Again, the primary goal is the patient's stability. This means reestablishing control of the diabetes, looking after the patient's emotional well-being, preventing infection, and promoting the healing of the surgical wound.

Usually, because the stress of surgery is diminished postoperatively, the insulin requirements also decrease — especially if a source of infection was removed. But if the patient is still stressed and anxious, and particularly if the surgery has altered his body image or confirmed a diagnosis that could change his life-style, insulin requirements probably won't decrease, and they might even increase. Each individual's coping mechanisms are different.

Your nursing care of the patient will include:
- checking and evaluating the vital signs
- measuring intake and output
- checking dressings for drainage
- monitoring all tubes for patency and function
- conscientiously observing I.V. infusions
- accurately recording all the above data
- taking fractional urines and checking blood glucose, if ordered.

In addition, observe your patient carefully for signs of either impending diabetic coma or diabetic ketoacidosis (DKA), which result from too little insulin; or hypoglycemia or insulin reaction, which result from too much insulin.

DKA may come not only from insufficient natural insulin or an inadequate or omitted insulin dosage but also from acute illness or medications such as cortisone that similarly raise the blood glucose levels. Since the metabolic derangement here is hyperglycemia, the treatment is insulin.

Hypoglycemia or insulin reaction results not only from too much insulin but also from omission or delay of meals, too much exercise without supportive food intake, or nutritional and fluid imbalances from nausea and vomiting. Excessive nausea and vomiting can also lead to DKA.

But up to a certain point, an insulin reaction is the more dangerous of these two complications. If severe enough, or if habitual, it can leave the patient who survives it with brain damage expressed as loss of memory, diminished ability to learn, or even paralysis. The central nervous system is acutely sensitive to glucose deprivation. When blood glucose levels are high, as in ketoacidosis, the brain can still use available glucose even in the absence of insulin. But when blood glucose levels are low, the brain is altogether robbed of the glucose it must have. Many doctors consider consistently spilling a little glucose into the urine preferable to too narrow a line of control with its risk of hypoglycemia.

After Angela S. had been returned to her room following her cystoscopic examination, her nurse noticed that she seemed more than ordinarily sleepy for a patient out of anesthesia for several hours. The nurse put her hand on the patient's forehead and asked her how she felt. She received a rather drunken-sounding reply and felt perspiration on Angela's forehead.

It turned out that the extra regular insulin given that morning

Watch out for infections
Infections (especially staphylococcal and mixed gram-negative) are a grave problem among diabetic patients. During and after surgery the patient may undergo derangements of nervous system function so that he loses sensation in infected areas. Remember that you can't count on pain to warn you about infection, so watch closely for minor lesions that could become serious problems if unattended.

to control her hyperglycemia had thrown her into a slight re-action. If such a patient can be aroused, 4 oz of orange juice will offset this reaction.

The treatment for insulin reaction is sugar, given quickly. If your patient is awake, give 4 oz of orange juice, two sugar lumps, or two teaspoons of honey as a starting dose — 10 g of carbohydrates altogether. Sometimes, you'll need to start I.V. glucose even with patients who are still awake. The treat-ment for those already in coma is usually 20 to 50 ml of 50% intravenous glucose given by push. For those patients not in shock so long that their available liver glycogen stores have been exhausted, glucagon may be ordered.

When the insulin-shock patient recovers, the cause needs to be found. It may mean reassessing his program.

These are the two sides of diabetes, then: two extreme derangements leading to coma and ultimate death if untreated, and two opposite treatments. Yet superficially, the two derangements may resemble each other. What of the confu-sion? Remember, whereas glucose given to a DKA patient even in coma need not spell the difference between life and death that minute, *insulin can kill a shock patient.*

Whenever there is a question between insulin hypoglycemia (shock) and DKA, always give the patient *glucose.* If it turns out to be DKA, little harm will have been done. If it is insulin shock, you will probably have saved a life!

Pending laboratory tests, what is the best way to check these patients for either threat? When the patient is sleeping, check for warm, dry skin and smell his breath for a *sweet, fruity odor* — that would be DKA. It is often accompanied by *fast, labored breathing* — a respiratory compensation for the met-abolic acidosis.

Check for *diaphoresis* by touching his gown and pillow case; dampness would mean hypoglycemia. This may also be accompanied by nightmares or sleepwalking. If you wonder whether the patient is actually asleep or progressing quietly into coma, don't hesitate to awaken him.

And other nursing measures are special to the patient with diabetes mellitus. His susceptibility to infection, for example, means you should encourage him to breathe deeply in order to minimize the possibility of pneumonia. Use scrupulous asepsis when catheterizing such a patient, caring for the cath-eters, or changing his dressing.

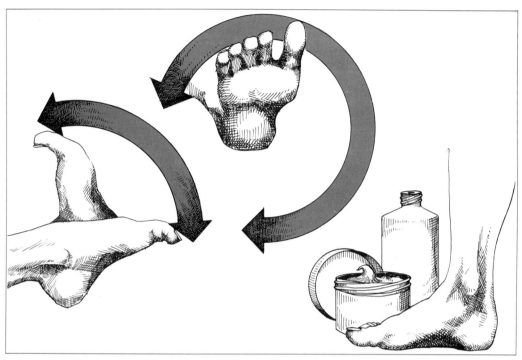

Premature peripheral vascular disease is another threat to the diabetic patient. Be doubly alert to any signs and symptoms of developing thrombophlebitis. Encourage the patient to turn and move to prevent decubiti and to exercise his legs to prevent pulmonary emboli. Elevating the legs and wearing elastic support hose also help prevent thrombophlebitis. The hose should be removed every 8 hours and the skin examined for redness and pressure sores. Keep his skin clean and dry, and *never* use ordinary adhesive tape on it.

Further management of the metabolism. Oral calorie intake is practically always preferable to intravenous feedings in a diabetic patient. As soon as possible after surgery, feed him and record the calories consumed. A progression to his usual diabetic diet will get him back on his normal regulated insulin dosage.

For the diabetic patient with postoperative or preoperative nasogastric suction, be on your guard against acidosis, electrolyte imbalance, dehydration, and starvation. Carefully record the amounts of I.V. solutions given so as to calibrate the glucose calories the patient receives.

For the patient on hyperalimentation, regular insulin is usually calculated and given to fit each patient's need. This need

Exercise even when ill
Bedridden diabetic patients must exercise to help circulation in their legs. They should extend and flex, abduct and adduct each foot at least 10 times a day. If feet are dry, they should apply lanolin or cocoa butter to prevent cracking and lesions.

is determined by blood glucose levels and by the total number of calories being administered. If the hyperalimentated or, indeed, any diabetic patient has a blood glucose level greater than 240 mg/dl, look for sepsis that might be causing the hyperglycemia. Check cultures of urine and blood. Examine the area where the tubing is inserted and the tubing itself. Check the clinical signs and the patient's general well-being. The increase in blood glucose levels should be covered with regular insulin.

Be sure that your diabetic surgical patient is adequately hydrated. If he is protected against hypoglycemic shock by continuous mild hyperglycemia, then polyuria and gradual dehydration are a chronic threat. If they continue unchecked over a period, this could add up to another metabolic crisis: hyperglycemic hyperosmolar nonketotic coma. Treatment, rather than depending on insulin, stresses the replacement of the vast quantities of liquid wasted by the osmotic diuresis.

Teaching. Even though the patient may have had diabetes mellitus for several years, there may be gaps in his understanding of it and perhaps room for improvement in his carrying out his own regimen. Teach your diabetic patient whatever you can, and teach his family, too. A dietary consult well in advance of discharge may be helpful. Document your teaching plan.

When he is ready to leave, you may want to refer him to a community health agency or to some community health personnel. The doctor will decide what his regimen is, but your place in helping him understand it and carry it out can be critical.

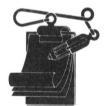

Remember these important points about avoiding the diabetes-related ill effects of surgery:
1. Realize that the stress of surgery releases ACTH from the pituitary; this increased stress eventually raises blood glucose levels, requiring more insulin.
2. Be aware that how you prepare your patient for surgery usually depends on your patient's diabetic regimen and the doctor's method of choice.
3. If you must add insulin to the patient's I.V., add only regular insulin to avoid delayed reactions.
4. Following surgery, aim to reestablish control of the patient's diabetes: look after his emotional well-being, prevent infection, and promote surgical wound healing.

18

Getting ready for medical tests

BY CATHERINE GAROFANO, RN, BS

GIVEN THE SERIOUS NATURE of major surgery and illnesses and the changeable nature of diabetes, you'd expect a very ill or surgical diabetic patient to challenge all your nursing skills. The last chapter certainly confirmed your expectations.

But what would you expect with a diabetic patient undergoing a simple diagnostic procedure, such as a gastric analysis or an upper GI series? True, the nursing protocol may not be as intricate. But it's every bit as important as the protocol for a surgical diabetic patient. Because just a simple slip-up in your preparation or instructions can send the patient headlong into hypoglycemia or hyperglycemia and even ketoacidosis.

Consider, for example, Calvin Brown, an inpatient who was sent to the lab for a routine gastric analysis. Because he was scheduled for his test at 10 a.m. and was to be NPO beforehand, the floor nurse assumed she should withhold his usual insulin dose. The lab was backed up with patients, so Calvin waited…and waited. After 1½ hours, he began to feel tired, weak, and thirsty. When he began complaining of stomach cramps, the lab technicians called his unit. Fortunately the head nurse recognized the symptoms as hyperglycemia with possible ketoacidosis and ordered Calvin returned to the unit without delay. She contacted the doctor for orders to treat the hyperglycemia. Then she talked to the nurse on Calvin's unit and explained that because Calvin's appointment was so late in the morning, she should have asked the doctor about giving him part of his insulin and a slow drip of I.V. glucose to maintain blood glucose control before and during the test. Or better yet, she should have had the test rescheduled for 7 a.m. so Calvin could stick to his normal routine.

Adhering to such simple guidelines will help you keep patients like Calvin Brown poised in diabetic balance before and after diagnostic tests. Here's a brief review.

No matter what
An insulin-dependent patient requires his insulin whether he eats or not. If he hasn't eaten, though, the dosage should be adjusted — to account not only for the lack of food but also for his hormonal milieu. As you'll remember from the last chapter, stressful situations, such as diagnostic tests, stimulate the production of certain hormones, such as cortisol and epinephrine. These insulin antagonists in turn increase the body's insulin needs. So insulin dosages must be carefully calculated.

If at all possible, procedures for insulin-dependent diabetic patients should be performed first thing in the morning. That way, the patient will be able to take food and his usual insulin dose in the morning after he returns from the test.

With radiologic procedures (such as a GI series, barium enema, or intravenous pyelogram [IVP]) your hospital may have you give the patient only clear liquids or a simple carbohydrate diet the evening before the test. In planning for his meal and a bedtime snack, take care to check the caloric needs of a patient on an intermediate insulin and to order foods that will cover them adequately.

The doctor must adjust the evening dose of insulin for patients who normally receive insulin both in the morning and in the evening. Watch these patients carefully through the night for signs of possible reactions — either hypoglycemia or hyperglycemia. Test their blood or urine for glucose every 4 to 6 hours; give a liquid sugar, such as orange juice, or an injection of glucose or glucagon followed by an I.V. drip of dextrose 5% in water to counteract hypoglycemia, and a small dose of regular insulin as ordered by the doctor to counteract hyperglycemia.

The patient should be kept NPO the morning of the procedure. Some hospitals suggest that you withhold the morning dose of insulin until the patient has returned from the procedure and can eat. If this is standard in your hospital and the patient will probably miss one meal that day, reduce his insulin dose. A better approach when possible, though, is to give the patient half of his usual morning dose at the usual time and start him on an I.V. drip of dextrose 5% in water at the rate of 1,000 ml/8 hours. Continue the I.V. through the procedure. Afterward, discontinue the I.V. Give the patient a small morning meal and the remainder of his insulin dose.

But if your patient's scheduled for an IVP, check with the radiologist before starting the I.V. Some radiologists believe the I.V. infusion dilutes the dye in the kidney and prefer performing the test first thing in the morning instead of starting an infusion.

Remember these important points about getting a diabetic patient ready for medical tests:
1. Keep in mind that an insulin-dependent diabetic patient requires insulin whether he eats or not.
2. If your patient hasn't eaten, adjust the dosage to account for the lack of food and his hormonal status.
3. If possible, arrange diagnostic procedures for insulin-dependent diabetic patients in the morning.
4. On the morning of the procedure, give your patient half his usual dose of insulin at the usual time and start him on an I.V. drip of dextrose 5% in water at the rate of 1,000 ml/8 hours, continuing the I.V. throughout the procedure.
5. Because an I.V. infusion may dilute dye concentration, check with the radiologist before starting one in a patient scheduled for an IVP.

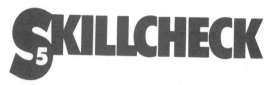

SKILLCHECK
5

1. Elliot Martin, 52 years old with IDDM, has gone into the hospital for excision of a benign tumor. Even though he knows the tumor is benign and the surgery is minor, Mr. Martin seems very nervous about the operation. He hasn't been eating well so he tells you to decrease his insulin dose. What would you tell him?

2. Francine Wilkes and Robert Upshaw, both diabetic patients, are on your medical-surgical unit awaiting surgery. A nursing student asks if you have a standard set of nursing rules for diabetic surgical patients. You tell her that care for diabetic patients has to be individualized. What five criteria would you use to individualize care for diabetic patients?

3. Michael MacDonnald, who controls his diabetes with Tolinase, is having outpatient diagnostic tests. He was scheduled for a 7 a.m. barium enema X-ray but, as usual, the radiology department is running behind schedule. Now, at 11:30 you find him in the hall still waiting for his X-ray. He seems very distracted, irritable, and shaky. What would you suspect?

4. Saul Jaffe, a diabetic patient usually controlled on oral agents, has been comatose from a stroke for 36 hours. Why must you test his blood for glucose and his urine for ketone every 1 to 6 hours?

5. Ron Kominsky, who normally takes 26 units of NPH insulin every morning, is scheduled for a prostatectomy at 7:00 this morning. You're in charge of preparing him for surgery. What orders would the doctor give you?

6. Adele Wister, age 54, controls her diabetes with 500 mg of Dymelor every morning. She is in the hospital now for a hysterectomy. To control her diabetes during hospitalization, the doctor has switched her to 8 units of regular insulin twice a day. After surgery, you check her blood for glucose and urine for ketone every 6 hours. In her latest urine test, you find that she is spilling ketones. She is sweating profusely and sleeping fitfully. When you try to rouse her, she doesn't respond. What should you do?

(Answers begin on page 208)

SKILLCHECK ANSWERS

ANSWERS TO SKILLCHECK 1

Situation 1 — Morton O'Reilly
No. During his hospitalization, Mr. O'Reilly has been unusually sedentary, eating a special diet, and under a great deal of stress. All of these conditions could skew his blood glucose levels. He should have a repeat fasting blood glucose test and a 2-hour postprandial glucose test at one of his follow-up visits in a month or two.

Situation 2 — Willard Jones
No. Glucose values rise with age. Mr. Jones' glucose tolerance test would almost certainly be abnormal if interpreted by conventional criteria designed for generally healthy young adults; norms for elderly people aren't available. Instead of a glucose tolerance test, Mr. Jones might have a 2-hour postprandial glucose determination. (Results below 225 mg/dl would be normal; results above 225 mg/dl could indicate a need for therapy, probably dietary adjustments.)

Situation 3 — Martha Simon
You could suggest two alternatives and let Ms. Simon take her pick. On her active days, she could eat a midmorning snack of a slow-acting carbohydrate (crackers or bread) followed by a snack of protein or fat. If her weight is normal and she has no trouble maintaining it, she would probably choose this alternative since her activity would burn off the additional calories. If Ms. Simon is overweight and is struggling to lose pounds, however, she might prefer to decrease her insulin dose on active days. To determine a realistic dose of insulin for active days, have her check her blood glucose levels before lunch on those particular days.

Situation 4 — Julie
One piece of fruit, which is a fast-acting carbohydrate, usually won't control an insulin-dependent diabetic patient's glucose level for long. Julie should have a slower-acting carbohydrate with protein or fat to better control her nocturnal glucose levels. You might suggest crackers and cheese. If Julie doesn't want to increase her caloric intake, you could suggest that she decrease her dinner by a bread and meat exchange and then eat these later as a bedtime snack. Reducing her intake at dinner will improve her bedtime Clinitest results, and eating a bedtime snack will maintain her glucose levels through the night.

Situation 5 — Paul
Extreme hunger often signals elevated blood glucose levels. Paul appears to be caught on the treadmill of eating more food, leading to a higher blood glucose level, leading to increased urinary loss of glucose, leading to more hunger, leading to more eating. His rapid growth during adolescence also may have altered his insulin needs. To ensure Paul's full growth potential during adolescence, you must stabilize his diabetes. Paul may need to be hospitalized briefly to establish dietary control. Then, you can help him realistically evaluate his total caloric intake. Paul may not fit into the standard dietary guidelines and may find a high-calorie diet with substantial snacks better suited to his life-style and needs.

Situation 6 — Harold Jefferson
Mr. Jefferson is a poor candidate for oral hypoglycemic agents for two reasons. First, he is taking hydrochlorothiazide, a thiazide diuretic that may provoke hyperglycemia. In fact, he might find that his blood glucose levels would fall considerably if he switched to a different diuretic. Second, he also has cardiac problems; some studies have shown that oral agents, particularly the sulfonylureas, increase the risk of death from cardiac disease. Still, Mr. Jefferson could use oral agents if he were changed to another type of diuretic that wouldn't affect his blood glucose and if his doctor felt that oral therapy were best for Mr. Jefferson despite his cardiac problems. Allergy to one sulfa drug often indicates allergy to all sulfa and sulfa-like drugs. But remember, Mr. Jefferson is allergic to sulfisoxazole. So chances are he'd be allergic to sulfonylureas, which are chemically related to sulfonamide antimicrobial drugs. Be sure to find out what type of reaction he had to sulfa.

Situation 7 — Jane Scarlotti
Ms. Scarlotti may not be responding as well to tolbutamide today as when she started the drug 5 years ago for two reasons. First, her compliance may be below par. Her forgetfulness about taking the drug may occur more frequently than she admits. Second, Ms. Scarlotti may be experiencing secondary failure to sulfonylurea, which sometimes occurs after several years of good diabetic control. The doctor may consider changing to a newer second-generation sulfonylurea, such as glyburide or glipizide. Many patients who develop secondary failure to the first-generation drug respond well when a second-generation drug is sub-

stituted. Also, tolbutamide is a first-generation sulfonylurea and should be taken twice daily; glyburide and
glipizide need be taken only once daily so Ms. Scarlotti's compliance may improve.

Situation 8 — Sarah Steinman
There are several likely reasons for Ms. Steinman's
variable response to insulin. She may be alternating
the order of her insulins when she draws them up,
causing variations in the mixture because of dead
space. To ensure a constant response, she should
draw up the insulins in the same order every day. Or,
if she has periodic local reactions to injections, such
as edema, absorption of the insulin may be delayed.
This could account for the hypoglycemic reaction if
she isn't getting food at the right time to counteract
the insulin's initial impact. Or, Ms. Steinman may not
be adjusting her insulin dose to coincide with variations
in her level of activity or stress. Finally, she may have
used contaminated or deteriorated insulin. Remind her
to discard any "suspicious" insulin.

Situation 9 — Frank Fisher
You should explain to the student that oral hypoglycemic therapy is always a risk in hospitalized patients.
The stress of hospitalization to the patient plus dietary
changes in the hospital often cause glucose levels to
fluctuate considerably. Oral hypoglycemic agents can't
control diabetes under these conditions. So, the patient should be switched to insulin during his hospital
stay.

Situation 10 — Jacqueline Bond
If Ms. Bond will be eating a large lunch on some days,
she should eat something on other days to establish
consistency. She can obtain her carbohydrates, proteins, and fats in a quick meal, such as a hamburger,
fruit, and perhaps potato chips or french fries. She
should have her lunch calculated as both a full-course
meal and as a quick meal. As for the cocktails at business lunches, Ms. Bond can accommodate the alcohol
by lowering her fat consumption at lunch. Once Ms.
Bond establishes a consistent diet, she may need to
adjust her insulin to account for the changes in her
eating habits.

ANSWERS TO SKILLCHECK 2

Situation 1 — Frank Melton
The elevation in Mr. Melton's urine glucose level after

supper and throughout the night may be caused simply
by poor dietary habits. He may be eating an excessively large dinner or bedtime snack, which his insulin
can't accommodate. If dietary control doesn't correct
the problem, though, Mr. Melton could add an intermediate or long-acting insulin to his morning dose of
insulin. That would give him better 24-hour control. If
that doesn't work, though, he could take a small dose
of intermediate insulin before dinner to guarantee overnight control.

Situation 2 — Gretchen Hanson
There are two potential errors in Gretchen's technique.
First, she says she "shakes" the bottle. If that's true,
she may be creating air bubbles or foam in the bottle,
which would prevent her from drawing up an accurate
dosage. You should remind her that she should mix
the insulin *gently* by inverting the bottle a few times.
Second, Gretchen doesn't say that she checks the
syringe for air bubbles or tries to eliminate them. Remind her to look for them and to remove them by pulling
the plunger back and then pushing it in to the correct
number of units, by flicking the barrel of the syringe
with her finger, or by pushing the insulin back into the
bottle and drawing up another dose.

Of course, Gretchen also may be slipping off her
diet or may simply need a change in dosage.

One more error in Gretchen's technique bears men-
tioning, even though it wouldn't affect her dosage: She
doesn't say that she washed her hands before starting
an injection. Be sure to remind her how important this
step is, since diabetic patients are susceptible to infections.

Situation 3 — Bill Preston
Mr. Preston will be on the plane about 8 hours, so he
should take along a snack of crackers in case he experiences a hypoglycemic reaction. Since less than
24 hours will elapse between his insulin injection at
home and his next injection in Paris, he probably should
take a much smaller dose of regular insulin and a somewhat smaller dose of NPH insulin in Paris; his doctor
can tell him exactly how much less to take. On subsequent mornings in Paris, he will take his usual dose.
When returning, since less than 24 hours will elapse
again, he should follow the same protocol he followed
on the trip over.

Situation 4 — Jill Collins
First, tell Jill that she should eat something. If she can't

eat a normal diet, she should try to substitute the foods recommended for an insulin-dependent diabetic patient — ginger ale, soup, and the like. Liquids are particularly important to replace fluids lost in diarrhea. Since Jill has already taken her Orinase this morning, she must eat something today to prevent hypoglycemia. However, if she absolutely can't eat anything on subsequent days, she should stop taking her Orinase during those days.

Situation 5 — Pat
Congratulate Pat on the negative results. Be sure to ask her if she's following her diet and getting adequate exercise. Find out if she's taking the same insulin dose.

Situation 6 — Randy Thomas
Randy is experiencing symptoms of hyperglycemia in the afternoon, so his urine test results probably would be low before breakfast and lunch, very high before dinner, and somewhat reduced (though still high) before his bedtime snack. This pattern indicates either that Randy is eating way too much at lunch and in the afternoon, or that he isn't taking enough intermediate insulin to see him through the afternoon and evening. In either case, he should be very concerned because this pattern could develop into ketoacidosis if uncorrected. Randy can correct the problem by sticking to his prescribed diet or by slightly increasing the dose of his Lente insulin, depending on his preference and his doctor's suggestion.

Situation 7 — Marvin Kissinger
Basically, Mr. Kissinger should simply stick to his usual diet and enjoy himself. Since German cooking often contains starchy vegetables, however, he should keep careful count of his carbohydrate intake. If he will be drinking ale or beer, he should eliminate 1½ bread exchanges for each 8-oz glass. Dry wine is permissible with dinner, if taken in small quantities.

ANSWERS TO SKILLCHECK 3

Situation 1 — Frank Masullo
The doctor is checking for fatty accumulation beneath the skin, caused by repeated injections in the same site. Mr. Masullo may be using the same injection sites over and over because they've become fibrous and less sensitive. By using fibrous sites, though, Mr. Masullo isn't getting the full effect of his insulin, since fibrous areas absorb poorly.

Situation 2 — Edwin Allen
Based on Mr. Allen's confused, almost drunken behavior, you should suspect insulin-induced hypoglycemia. Mr. Allen may have compromised cerebral function due to his age and cerebral arteriosclerosis.

Any slight decline in his blood glucose level would further impair his reasoning abilities, so that he might not recognize the early symptoms of hypoglycemia. The time of day may be another clue to Mr. Allen's condition. He would be most likely to experience hypoglycemia in the late afternoon, since his NPH insulin would peak then. Mr. Allen may have skipped lunch and not have enough glucose to balance the insulin. Remember, too, that patients taking intermediate or long-acting insulin don't always show the classic symptoms of hypoglycemia. These insulins cause a slow decline in blood glucose levels, making cerebral symptoms more pronounced. Aphasia, uncoordinated movements, and psychotic behavior are common.

Situation 3 — Margaret Morris
Chances are Ms. Morris is in an ICU. Her condition is acute and demands constant attention, particularly attention to her blood glucose level and her fluid intake and output. The first step in treatment would be to correct the insulin deficiency with I.V. insulin and to correct the dehydration, sodium depletion, and low blood volume with an I.V. of normal saline solution. After urinary output and renal blood flow were stabilized, she would receive I.V. potassium to correct the electrolyte imbalance and glucose to prevent her condition from going to the other extreme, hypoglycemia. But fluid output would have to be carefully monitored for adequate output before potassium could be added to the I.V. If output isn't adequate, the patient probably is retaining potassium; added potassium could cause dangerous cardiac dysrhythmias.

Situation 4 — Andrew Sims
Don't be deceived by the fruity smell on Mr. Sims' breath. Although fruity breath and flushing may be consistent with DKA, four vital symptoms — strong pulse, profuse sweating, dilated pupils, and confusion and disorientation — point strongly to hypoglycemia. The fruity smell on Mr. Sims' breath could be alcohol or something else he had eaten. And the flushing may simply be Mr. Sims' individual way of responding to hypoglycemia. A blood glucose test would probably be negative, confirming hypoglycemia.

Situation 5 — Jamie
The elevated blood glucose level without accompanying ketones indicates HHNC. Jamie probably already had diabetes before he developed the throat infection. The infection increased his need for insulin, though, making his endogenous supply inadequate. Fever and vomiting contributed to Jamie's dehydration. Stress, insulin deficiency, and dehydration all combined to produce hyperglycemia. When superimposed on Jamie's preexisting diabetes, the hyperglycemia became exaggerated and turned into HHNC.

Situation 6 — Anne Loomis

Chances are her visual difficulties are only transitory. Anne is young and has just recently developed diabetes, so the possibility of permanent eye damage from her diabetes, such as retinopathy, is remote. Many diabetic patients have trouble with their vision until their diabetes is stabilized because the accumulation of sorbital and fructose in the lens causes the eye to swell. When the glucose level returns to normal, the lens returns to its original shape and vision often improves.

Tell Anne that this process may take 6 to 8 weeks after she begins therapy. However, she should consult her doctor now to make sure she doesn't have any serious difficulty, such as a detached retina.

Situation 7 — George Franklin

Extensive dermatitis resembles burns in that the loss of skin integrity in both conditions results in an increased secretion of endogenous glucocorticoids. In Mr. Franklin's case, that natural process has been aggravated by high doses of exogenous steroids. The excess glucocorticoids have probably undercut his endogenous insulin's ability to metabolize glucose, resulting in hyperglycemia. If the glucocorticoids also suppressed release of ADH, osmotic diuresis probably led to dehydration. Mr. Franklin's I.V. fluids weren't enough to prevent dehydration. What's more, the fluids contain carbohydrates that would worsen his hyperglycemia. Although Mr. Franklin is receiving Lente insulin, it probably isn't enough to metabolize the glucose: thus, the HHNC. To lower his blood glucose level, give a supplement of regular insulin.

Situation 8 — Vicki James

Actually, Vicki doesn't need her emergency kit. She could easily take 10 g of carbohydrate — for instance, 3 oz of cola or five or six hard candies — to correct her hypoglycemia. But if she must choose from her kit, she should select the dextrose wafer. (Glucagon, Glutose and epinephrine all should be reserved for more advanced hypoglycemia.) Whether she uses a common carbohydrate or the dextrose wafer, though, she should follow it with a slower-acting carbohydrate, such as peanut butter or bread. This combination will stem her immediate hypoglycemic reaction while providing ongoing glucose coverage.

ANSWERS TO SKILLCHECK 4

Situation 1 — Johnny Stover

Because he'll be getting more exercise than usual on his baseball days, Johnny will have to supplement his usual diet. Since he's a growing child, he should have more food at his noon meal and afternoon snack. He also should take a simple sugar to baseball practice in case he misjudges the food-insulin balance and becomes hypoglycemic. Johnny also should delay his evening insulin injection until he's free from practice and ready for supper. But he shouldn't decrease his insulin dose; otherwise, he might not have adequate control throughout the night. Although Johnny should be able to manage his diabetes with these adjustments, he also should make sure the coach or some other responsible adult with the team knows about his condition and can recognize all the signs of hypoglycemia. That person should keep hard candy or cola on hand and know when to administer them.

Situation 2 — Mary Willis

Mrs. Willis has every right to be concerned about Mary's blood glucose results. Severe hypoglycemia, of course, could cause irreversible brain damage. Still, Mrs. Willis seems to be overly concerned about the results. You should try to give her a more positive outlook on diabetes. Explain again the relationship of food and insulin to glucose levels and that proper therapy will keep Mary out of danger. If Mary refuses to eat exactly the foods on her meal plan, show her how to make substitutions from exchange lists. Also make sure she knows how to adjust food to coincide with activity levels. Finally, make sure she knows how to treat hypoglycemia with a high-glucose food or with glucagon. Mrs. Willis' anxiety will probably ease as she becomes more accustomed to the idea of Mary's diabetes and more proficient at caring for her. In the meantime, you could introduce her to well-adjusted mothers of other diabetic children; perhaps they could help her see Mary's diabetes as manageable.

Situation 3 — Terry

Try to get her to see her diabetes not as an illness but as a condition that simply needs to be controlled. Ask her to explain why she feels this way about her diabetes. If possible, arrange a group meeting with other diabetic teenagers or introduce Terry individually to other diabetic teenagers. If they have adjusted to their disease, they may change Terry's perspective; or, if they are having a similar reaction, simply talking it over may help both of them. You also might suggest consultation with a psychiatric nurse, if one is available. The important step here is to get Terry to express her feelings. If she doesn't, she may stage a quiet rebellion by simply ignoring her diabetic therapy.

Situation 4 — Debby Rosen

From every indication, Debby can expect a normal, happy pregnancy, with little risk to herself or the baby. Debby qualifies as a Class C diabetic patient. She could develop hydramnios, toxemia, or urinary tract infections, as could any pregnant diabetic patient. But the chances are slight if she follows the doctor's orders and gets a checkup every 2 weeks; even if the conditions do develop, they can be treated. Since Debby is already managing her diabetes well with insulin, she won't have to change her therapy except to make minor adjustments in her insulin dose and diet to meet her changing needs throughout her pregnancy. The critical time of her pregnancy will occur after the 30th week; but the doctor will see her more often then and check her estriol level weekly to determine the best time for delivery. If all goes well, he'll probably deliver by cesarean section in the 36th or 37th week.

Situation 5 — Ed Phillips
Reassure Mr. Phillips that many blind diabetic patients live alone and do it quite well. Teach him how to measure his insulin injections and administer them; you might suggest some injection devices, such as the copper sleeve, to help him guarantee accurate dose measurement. With some vision in his right eye, Mr. Phillips may be able to see when his insulin vials are empty. To be on the safe side, though, he should follow the practice of totally blind diabetic patients and use marbles to count doses. Mr. Phillips also may have enough vision to test his urine using color strips. If not, you should teach him the yeast method of testing urine. If Mr. Phillips won't be able to cook for himself, refer him to a local service agency, such as Meals on Wheels, an agency for the blind, or a local diabetes group. If none of these is available, you could help him arrange to dine with friends or at restaurants on a regular basis and to prepare simple meals at home.

Situation 6 — Eileen Shaunnessy
You could recommend any of several devices to help with self-injections. Many visually impaired diabetic patients prefer the Insulgage loading gauge because they can use it to vary dosages and to measure mixed doses. But if Ms. Shaunnessy must use a glass syringe for economic reasons, she might do better using the copper sleeve, which is designed specifically for a reusable syringe. If she uses U-100 insulin and seldom varies the dose, she might prefer a Hill accurate dose syringe. Find out which devices best meet her specific needs. To remove air bubbles, Ms. Shaunnessy should draw up the insulin three times before injecting. If Ms. Shaunnessy still feels uneasy about giving herself injections, suggest that she have a nurse — friend, neighbor, or visiting nurse — check on her periodically.

Situation 7 — Nancy Byers
Advise Nancy to see her diabetologist right away. Stopping her oral hypoglycemic agent at this point might do more harm than good because, without it, her diabetes will be completely uncontrolled. That, of course, could be very harmful to the fetus. But the doctor will change Nancy to insulin for the duration of her pregnancy and during lactation.

Situation 8 — Ted Nichols
Ted can adjust to the trip quite easily if he makes these simple adjustments: plans to eat extra food to cover his insulin dose during extra activity, or, if he can't tolerate the extra food, cuts his insulin dose slightly. He should also carry a simple sugar with him in case he experiences hypoglycemic reactions. To be on the safe side, Ted should travel with someone who knows of his condition and can recognize and treat hypoglycemic reactions. He should always carry glucagon.

Situation 9 — Susan Hendricks
No. Clinitest results are unreliable during lactation because lactose spills into the urine, causing a false-positive reading. Suggest that she get some Tes-Tape for urine testing; it tests specifically for glucose. If Tes-Tape results are positive, have her contact her doctor for further instructions.

ANSWERS TO SKILLCHECK 5

Situation 1 — Elliot Martin
Actually, Mr. Martin probably should increase his insulin dose. His anxiety coupled with the bodily insult of the surgery itself will have a diabetogenic effect. The sympathetic nervous system will release adrenocorticotropic hormone (ACTH) as well as the glucocorticoids of the adrenal cortex and epinephrine. Both ACTH and the glucocorticoids promote gluconeogenesis; epinephrine facilitates glycogenolysis. All of that results in an elevated blood glucose level, which requires more insulin. If Mr. Martin isn't eating, though, his blood glucose level may not rise much higher than his usual level. To determine exactly how much insulin he should take, you will have to check his urine every 4 to 6 hours.

Situation 2 — Francine Wilkes and Robert Upshaw
The five criteria are: severity of the diabetes, nature of the surgery, presence of diabetic complications, nondiabetic diagnosis, and the doctor's preference in treatment.

Severity of the diabetes depends on the age of onset, stage of diabetes, and usual method of control. Nature of the surgery means whether it is minor or major, elective or emergency. The labels "minor" and "major" depend not only on the amount of physical trauma but also on the length of the procedure, anesthetic used, and the patient's psychological reaction to the surgery. (What normally is considered minor surgery may be considered major for some patients because they react so strongly to it, creating great stress and greatly altering glucose metabolism. Local or spinal anesthetics cause fewer metabolic disturbances than a general anesthetic.)

Diabetic complications include hypertension, peripheral vascular disease, foot decubiti, or a gangrenous toe. The nondiabetic diagnosis refers to coexisting conditions, such as fistulae or cancer.

The doctor's treatment preference refers to his chosen method of controlling the patient's diabetes, based on all the above information.

Situation 3 — Michael MacDonnald

Mr. MacDonnald sounds as though he's having a hypoglycemic reaction. He probably was told not to eat before leaving home this morning, but he may have taken his Tolinase to cover his food intake later. Because he has had to wait so long without food, his blood glucose level has fallen below normal. You could confirm your suspicions with a quick blood glucose test. If his blood glucose level is low, you should give him a quick source of glucose (for example, hard candy or cola). He may have to reschedule his tests for another day. He could complete his test, however, if I.V. 50% glucose was given to increase his blood glucose level.

Situation 4 — Saul Jaffe

Even though Mr. Jaffe normally would qualify as mildly diabetic, in his present serious condition he must be treated as severely diabetic. He probably is receiving an I.V. of dextrose 5% in water and having his diabetes controlled with regular insulin every 6 hours. You must check his blood glucose level to determine whether he needs a larger or smaller dose. Mr. Jaffe probably has a Foley cathether. To obtain a specimen, do not disconnect the catheter. Instead, clamp the tubing for 15 to 30 minutes, allowing the urine to collect in the bladder. Then clean the tubing with an alcohol wipe and aspirate a small amount of urine using a 25G needle and syringe.

Situation 5 — Ron Kominsky

Since the surgery will be performed under a general anesthetic, you would keep Mr. Kominsky NPO the night before and the day of surgery. The doctor's orders would probably read as follows: 1 hour before the patient goes to the operating room, draw a stat blood glucose test. Then give one half to one third of his normal insulin dose subcutaneously and start an I.V. with dextrose 5% in water. If you are to administer a preoperative medication, such as morphine or Demerol, give only one half or three quarters the normal dose to avoid any nausea or vomiting. Nausea and vomiting could significantly lower his blood glucose level, upsetting his diabetic control.

Situation 6 — Adele Wister

Despite the ketones in her urine, Ms. Wister sounds as though she's going into hypoglycemic coma (restlessness, diaphoresis). The ketones in her urine could stem from an infection, dehydration, or drugs she is given. A stat blood glucose test will settle the question. But Ms. Wister also needs stat treatment. Give her an injection of glucagon right after you draw the stat blood. Remember that, when in doubt, you should give sugar to guard against the dire consequences of hypoglycemia.

Appendices

AMERICAN DIABETES ASSOCIATION
EXCHANGE DIET
All foods appearing in italics are low-fat or nonfat.

Free foods
There are certain foods you can use in unlimited amounts when planning your meals. Some of these include:

Diet calorie-free beverage	*Parsley*
Coffee	*Nutmeg*
Tea	*Lemon*
Bouillon without fat	*Mustard*
Unsweetened gelatin	*Chili powder*
Unsweetened pickles	*Onion salt or powder*
Salt and pepper	*Horseradish*
Red pepper	*Vinegar*
Paprika	*Mint*
Garlic	*Cinnamon*
Celery salt	*Lime*

Forbidden foods

Sugar	Jelly	Chewing gum
Candy	Cookies	Soft drinks
Honey	Syrup	Pies
Jam	Condensed milk	Cakes

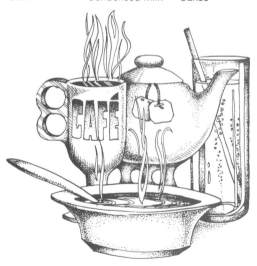

List one: Milk exchanges
One exchange of milk contains 12 g of carbohydrate, 8 g of protein, a trace of fat, and 80 calories. This list shows the kinds and amounts of milk or milk products to use for one milk exchange. Low-fat and whole milk contain saturated fat.

Nonfat fortified milk
Skim or nonfat milk . . . . 1 cup
Powdered (nonfat dry,
before adding liquid) . . . . ⅓ cup
Canned, evaporated skim milk . . . . ½ cup
Buttermilk made from skim milk . . . . 1 cup
Yogurt made from skim milk
(plain, unflavored) . . . . 1 cup
Low-fat fortified milk
1%-fat fortified milk
(omit one half fat exchange) . . . . 1 cup
2%-fat fortified milk
(omit one fat exchange) . . . . 1 cup
Yogurt made from 2%-fat fortified milk
(plain, unflavored)
(omit one fat exchange) . . . . 1 cup
Whole milk (omit two fat exchanges)
Whole milk . . . . 1 cup
Canned, evaporated whole milk . . . . ½ cup
Buttermilk made from whole milk . . . . 1 cup
Yogurt made from whole milk
(plain, unflavored) . . . . 1 cup

List two: Vegetable exchanges
One exchange of vegetables contains about 5 g of carbohydrate, 2 g of protein, and 25 calories. This list shows the kinds of vegetables to use for one vegetable exchange.

Asparagus . . . . ½ cup
Bean sprouts . . . . ½ cup
Beets . . . . ½ cup
Broccoli . . . . ½ cup
Brussels sprouts . . . . ½ cup
Cabbage . . . . ½ cup
Carrots . . . . ½ cup
Cauliflower . . . . ½ cup

Vegetable exchanges (continued)

Celery . . . . ½ cup
Cucumbers . . . . ½ cup
Eggplant . . . . ½ cup
Green pepper . . . . ½ cup
Greens:
    Beet . . . . ½ cup
    Chard . . . . ½ cup
    Collard . . . . ½ cup
    Dandelion . . . . ½ cup
    Kale . . . . ½ cup
    Mustard . . . . ½ cup
    Spinach . . . . ½ cup
    Turnip . . . . ½ cup
Mushrooms . . . . ½ cup
Okra . . . . ½ cup
Onions . . . . ½ cup
Rhubarb . . . . ½ cup
Rutabaga . . . . ½ cup
Sauerkraut . . . . ½ cup
String beans, green or yellow . . . . ½ cup
Summer squash . . . . ½ cup
Tomatoes . . . . ½ cup
Tomato juice . . . . ½ cup
Turnips . . . . ½ cup
Vegetable juice cocktail . . . . ½ cup
Zucchini . . . . ½ cup

The following raw vegetables may be used as desired:

Chicory   Lettuce
Chinese cabbage   Parsley
Endive   Radishes
Escarole   Watercress

(Starchy vegetables are in the bread exchange list.)

List three: Fruit exchanges

One exchange of fruit contains 10 g of carbohydrate and 40 calories. This list shows the kinds and amounts of fruits to use for one fruit exchange.

Apple . . . . 1 small
Apple juice . . . . ⅓ cup
Applesauce (unsweetened) . . . . ½ cup
Apricots, fresh . . . . 2 medium
Apricots, dried . . . . 4 halves
Banana . . . . ½ small
Berries
    Blackberries . . . . ½ cup
    Blueberries . . . . ½ cup
    Raspberries . . . . ½ cup
    Strawberries . . . . ¾ cup
Cherries . . . . 10 large
Cider . . . . ⅓ cup
Dates 2
Figs, fresh or dried 1
Grapefruit . . . . ½
Grapefruit juice . . . . ½ cup

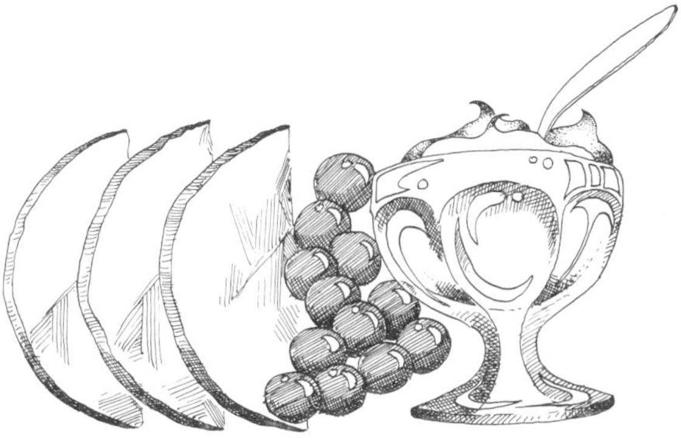

Grapes 12
Grape juice . . . . ¼ cup
Mango . . . . ½ small
Melon
    Cantaloupe . . . . ½ small
    Honeydew . . . . ⅛ medium
    Watermelon . . . . 1 cup
Nectarine . . . . 1 small
Orange . . . . 1 small
Orange juice . . . . ¼ cup
Papaya . . . . ¾ cup
Peach . . . . 1 medium
Pear . . . . 1 small
Persimmon, native . . . . 1 medium
Pineapple . . . . ½ cup
Pineapple juice . . . . ⅓ cup
Plums . . . . 2 medium
Prunes . . . . 2 medium
Prune juice . . . . ¼ cup
Raisins . . . . 2 tbs
Tangerine . . . . 1 medium

Cranberries may be used as desired if no sugar is added.

List four: Bread exchanges

One exchange of bread contains 15 g of carbohydrate, 2 g of protein, and 70 calories. This list shows the kinds and amounts of breads, cereals, starchy vegetables, and prepared foods to use for one bread exchange.

Cereal
    Bran flakes . . . . ½ cup
    Other ready-to-eat
       unsweetened cereal . . . . ¾ cup
    Puffed cereal (unfrosted) . . . . 1 cup
    Cereal (cooked) . . . . ½ cup
    Grits (cooked) . . . . ½ cup
    Rice or barley (cooked) . . . . ½ cup
    Pasta (cooked)
       Spaghetti, noodles,
       macaroni . . . . ½ cup

(Continued on next page)

Bread exchanges *(continued)*

Popcorn
  (popped, no fat added) . . . . 3 cups
Cornmeal (dry) . . . . 2 tbs
Flour . . . . 2½ tbs
Wheat germ . . . . ¼ cup
Crackers
  Graham, 2½" sq. 2
  Matzo, 4" × 6" . . . . ½
  Oyster 20
  Pretzels, 3⅛" long × ⅛" dia. 25
  Rye wafers, 2" × 3½" 3
  Saltines 6
  Soda, 2½" sq. 4
Dried beans, peas, and lentils
  Beans, peas, lentils
    (dried and cooked) . . . . ½ cup
  Baked beans, no pork
    (canned) . . . . ¼ cup
Starchy vegetables
  Corn . . . . ⅓ cup
  Corn on cob . . . . 1 small
  Lima beans . . . . ½ cup
  Parsnips . . . . ⅔ cup
  Peas, green (canned or frozen) . . . . ½ cup
  Potato, white . . . . 1 small
  Potato (mashed) . . . . ½ cup
  Pumpkin . . . . ¾ cup
  Winter squash,
    acorn or butternut . . . . ½ cup
  Yam or sweet potato . . . . ¼ cup
Prepared foods
  Biscuit, 2" dia.
    (omit one fat exchange) 1
  Corn bread, 2" × 2" × 1"
    (omit one fat exchange) 1
  Corn muffin, 2" dia.
    (omit one fat exchange) 1
  Crackers, round butter type
    (omit one fat exchange) 5
  Muffin, plain and small
    (omit one fat exchange) 1
  Potatoes, french fried,
    Length 2" to 3½"
    (omit one fat exchange) 8

Potato or corn chips
  (omit two fat exchanges) 15
Pancake, 5" × ½"
  (omit one fat exchange) 1
Waffle, 5" × ½"
  (omit one fat exchange) 1

List five: Meat exchanges
LEAN MEAT
One exchange of lean meat (1 oz) contains 7 g of protein, 3 g of fat, and 55 calories. This list shows the kinds and amounts of lean meat and other protein-rich foods to use for one low-fat meat exchange.
Beef:
  Baby beef (very lean), chipped beef,
  chuck, flank steak, tenderloin, plate ribs,
  plate skirt steak, round (bottom, top),
  all cuts rump, spare ribs, tripe . . . . 1 oz
Lamb:
  Leg, rib, sirloin, loin (roast and chops),
  shank, shoulder . . . . 1 oz
Pork:
  Leg (whole rump, center shank),
  ham, smoked (center slices) . . . . 1 oz
Veal:
  Leg, loin, rib, shank, shoulder,
  cutlets . . . . 1 oz
Poultry:
  Meat without skin of chicken, turkey,
  cornish hen, guinea hen,
  pheasant . . . . 1 oz
Fish:
  Any fresh or frozen . . . . 1 oz
  Canned salmon, tuna, mackerel, crab,
  lobster . . . . ¼ cup
  Clams, oysters, scallops,
  shrimp . . . . 5 or 1 oz
  Sardines, drained 3
Cheeses containing less than 5%
  butterfat . . . . 1 oz
Cottage cheese, dry and 2%
  butterfat . . . . ¼ cup
Dried beans and peas (omit one
  bread exchange) . . . . ½ cup

Meat exchanges *(continued)*

MEDIUM-FAT MEAT

For each exchange of medium-fat meat, omit one half fat exchange. This list shows the kinds and amounts of medium-fat meat and other protein-rich foods to use for one medium-fat meat exchange.

Beef:
 Ground (15% fat), corned beef (canned),
 rib eye, round (ground commercial) ....1 oz
Pork:
 Loin (all cuts tenderloin), shoulder arm
 (picnic), shoulder blade, Boston
 butt, Canadian bacon, boiled ham ....1 oz
Liver, heart, kidney, and sweetbreads
 (these are high in cholesterol) ....1 oz
Cottage cheese, creamed ....¼ cup
Cheese:
 Mozzarella, ricotta, farmer's cheese,
  neufchâtel ....1 oz
 Parmesan ....3 tbs
Egg (high in cholesterol) 1
Peanut butter (omit two additional
 fat exchanges) ....2 tbs

HIGH-FAT MEAT

For each exchange of high-fat meat, omit one fat exchange. This list shows the kinds and amounts of high-fat meat and other protein-rich foods to use for one high-fat meat exchange.

Beef:
 Brisket, corned beef (brisket), ground beef
 (more than 20% fat), hamburger (commercial),
 chuck (ground commercial), roasts (rib),
 steaks (club and rib) ....1 oz
Lamb:
 Breast ....1 oz
Pork:
 Spare ribs, loin (back ribs), pork (ground),
 country style ham, deviled ham ....1 oz
Veal:
 Breast ....1 oz
Poultry:
 Capon, duck (domestic), goose ....1 oz
Cheese:
 Cheddar types ....1 oz
Cold cuts ....4½" × ⅛" slice
Frankfurter ....1 small

List six: Fat exchanges

One exchange of fat contains 5 g of fat and 45 calories. This list shows the kinds and amounts of fat-containing foods to use for one fat exchange.

Margarine, soft, tub or stick* ....1 tsp
Avocado (4" dia.)† ....⅛

Oil
 Corn, cottonseed, safflower,
 soy, sunflower ....1 tsp
Oil, olive† ....1 tsp
Oil, peanut† ....1 tsp
Olives† ....5 small
Almonds† ....10 whole
Pecans† ....2 large
Peanuts†
 Spanish ....20 whole
 Virginia ....10 whole
Walnuts ....6 small
Nuts, other† ....6 small

Margarine, regular stick ....1 tsp
Butter ....1 tsp
Bacon fat ....1 tsp
Bacon, crisp ....1 strip
Cream, light ....2 tbs
Cream, sour ....2 tbs
Cream, heavy ....1 tbs
Cream cheese ....1 tbs
French dressing‡ ....1 tbs
Italian dressing‡ ....1 tbs
Lard ....1 tsp
Mayonnaise‡ ....1 tsp
Salad dressing, mayonnaise type‡ ....2 tsp
Salt pork ....¾" cube

*Made with corn, cottonseed, safflower, soy, or sunflower oil only
†Fat content is primarily monounsaturated
‡If made with corn, cottonseed, safflower, soy, or sunflower oil, can be used on fat-modified diet

DRUG INTERACTIONS WITH SULFONYLUREAS

INTERACTING DRUG	ORAL AGENTS	EFFECT
A		
acetazolamide (Diamox)	All	Hyperglycemia
alcohol	All	Hypoglycemia (acute ingestion only); hyperglycemia (chronic ingestion only); Antabuse-like reaction, especially with chlorpropamide
allopurinol (Zyloprim)	All	Hypoglycemia
anabolic steroid hormones (Adroyd*, Anavar*, Winstrol, etc.)	All	Hypoglycemia
aspirin	All	Hypoglycemia
B		
beta-adrenergic blockers	All	Hypoglycemia (without usual signs and symptoms)
bumetanide	All	Hyperglycemia
C		
chloramphenicol (Chloromycetin)	chlorpropamide, tolbutamide	Hypoglycemia
clofibrate (Atromid-S)	All	Hypoglycemia
corticosteroids (betamethasone, betamethasone valerate, cortisone, dexamethasone, hydrocortisone, triamcinolone acetonide, methylprednisolone, prednisolone, prednisone, etc.)	All	Hyperglycemia; corticosteroids impair glucose tolerance
D		
dextrothyroxine (Choloxin)	All	Hyperglycemia
diazoxide (Hyperstat)	All	Hyperglycemia; hypokalemia (replacement of potassium may return blood glucose to normal)

*Not available in Canada.

INTERACTING DRUG	ORAL AGENTS	EFFECT
dicumarol	All	Hypoglycemia; increased anticoagulant effect for several days followed by decreased anticoagulant effect
E		
epinephrine (Adrenalin, Sus-Phrine)	All	Hyperglycemia
ethacrynic acid (Edecrin)	All	Hyperglycemia
F		
fenfluramine	All	Hypoglycemia
furosemide (Lasix)	All	Hyperglycemia
G		
glucagon	All	Hyperglycemia
guanethidine (Ismelin)	All	Hypoglycemia
L		
levothyroxine (Synthroid)	All	Hyperglycemia
M		
marijuana	All	Hyperglycemia
methyldopa (Aldomet)	tolbutamide	Hypoglycemia
monoamine oxidase inhibitors (Eutonyl*, Marplan, Nardil, Parnate)	All	Hypoglycemia
O		
oxyphenbutazone (Oxalid*, Tandearil*)	All	Hypoglycemia
P		
phenothiazines (Compazine*, Mellaril, Phenergan, Prolixin*, Sparine, Stelazine, Temaril*, Thorazine*, etc.)	All	Hyperglycemia

*Not available in Canada.

(continued on next page)

DRUG INTERACTIONS WITH SULFONYLUREAS *(continued)*

INTERACTING DRUG	ORAL AGENTS	EFFECT
P		
phenylbutazone (Azolid*, Butazol-idin)	All	Hypoglycemia
phenytoin (Dilantin)	All	Hyperglycemia
probenecid (Benemid)	All	Hypoglycemia
R		
rifampin (Rifadin, Rimactane)	All	Hyperglycemia
S		
salicylates	All	Hypoglycemia
sulfinpyrazone	tolbutamide	Hypoglycemia
sulfonamides (Bactrim, Gantanol, Gantrisin, Septra, Thiosulfil)	All	Hypoglycemia
T		
thiazide diuretics (Diuril, Esidrix, HydroDIURIL, Oretic*, Renese, etc.)	All	Hyperglycemia; hypokalemia (replacement of potassium may return blood glucose to normal)
thyroid hormone	All	Hyperglycemia; increased thyroid effect

*Not available in Canada

Index

Selected References

Blevins, Dorothy. *The Diabetic and Nursing Care.* New York: McGraw-Hill Book Co., 1979.

Boden, G., et al. "Monitoring Metabolic Control in Diabetic Outpatients with Glycosylated Hemoglobin," *Annals of Internal Medicine* 92(3):357-60, March 1980.

Brownlee, Michael. "Achieving Better Blood Glucose Control," *Drug Therapy* 11(5):59-69, May 1981.

Childs, Belinda P. "Insulin Infusion Pumps: New Solution to an Old Problem," *Nursing83* 13:54-57, November 1983.

Davidson, Mayer B. *Diabetes Mellitus: Diagnosis and Treatment.* New York: John Wiley & Sons, 1981.

Espenshade, Jean, ed. *Staff Manual for Teaching Patients about Diabetes Mellitus.* Chicago: American Hospital Association, 1982.

Guthrie, Diana W., and Guthrie, Richard A. *Nursing Management of Diabetes Mellitus,* 2nd ed. St. Louis: C.V. Mosby Co., 1982.

Huff, T.A. "Exercise Planning for Insulin-Dependent Diabetics," *Consultant* 21:71-72, February 1981.

Israel, R.G., et al. "Exercise Effects on Fitness, Lipids, Glucose Tolerance, and Insulin Levels in Young Adults," *Archives of Physical Medicine and Rehabilitation* 62(7):336-41, July 1981.

Kintzel, Kay C., ed. *Advanced Concepts in Clinical Nursing,* 2nd ed. Philadelphia: J.B. Lippincott Co., 1977.

Levin, Marvin E., and O'Neal, Lawrence W. *The Diabetic Foot,* 3rd ed. St. Louis: C.V. Mosby Co., 1982.

McConnell, Edwina A. "Be Prepared for Double Trouble if Your Surgical Patient's a Diabetic," *Nursing81* 11:118-23, November 1981.

Nemchik, R. "Diabetes Today: Facing Up to Long-Term Complications," *RN* 46(7):38-45, July 1983.

Nemchik, R. "The New Insulin Pumps: Tight Control—At a Price," *RN* 46(5):52-59, May 1983.

Nyberg, Kathryne Gavin. "Diabetes Today: When Diabetes Complicates Your Pre- and Post-Op Care," *RN* 46:42-47, January 1983.

Peterson, C.M., ed. *Diabetes Management in the Nineteen Eighties: The Role of Home Blood Glucose Monitoring and New Insulin Delivery Systems.* New York: Praeger Publishers, 1982.

Podolsky, S. "Management of Diabetes in the Surgical Patient," *Medical Clinics of North America* 66(6):1361-72, November 1982.

Powers, D., et al. "Nursing Management of Diabetic Ketoacidosis," *Critical Care Quarterly* 3:139-43, September 1980.

Schiffrin, A., et al. "Improved Control in Diabetes with Continuous Subcutaneous Insulin Infusion," *Diabetes Care* 3:643-49, November/December 1980.

Schuler, K. "When a Pregnant Woman is Diabetic," Parts 1, 4. *American Journal of Nursing* 79:448-50 and 458-60, March 1979.

Steiner, George, and Lawrence, Patricia A. *Educating Diabetic Patients.* New York: Springer Publishing Co., 1981.